Guidelines
for
Graded Exercise Testing
and
Exercise Prescription

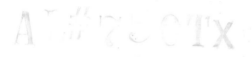

Guidelines
for
Graded Exercise Testing
and
Exercise Prescription

AMERICAN COLLEGE OF SPORTS MEDICINE

2nd Edition

Lea & Febiger   *Philadelphia*

Library of Congress Cataloging in Publication Data

American College of Sports Medicine.
    Guidelines for graded exercise testing and
exercise prescription.
     1. Exercise therapy. 2. Cardiovascular
patients—Rehabilitation. 3. Exercise tests.
I. Title. [DNLM: 1. Exercise test. 2. Exercise
therapy. 3. Exertion. WE103 A514g]
RC 684.E9A45 1980   615'.824   80-19484
ISBN 0-8121-0769-1

1st Edition, 1975
  Reprinted 1976
  Reprinted 1977
  Reprinted 1979
2nd Edition, 1980

PRINTED IN THE UNITED STATES OF AMERICA

Print number: 4   3

Preface

The impetus for the American College of Sports Medicine to undertake the writing and publication of the *Guidelines* originated at a special interest group meeting on Cardiac Rehabilitation at the Annual Meeting of the College held in Philadelphia in May, 1972. The recommendation from this meeting was that the College formulate a plan to assist the many new groups who were starting exercise programs. A special Sub-Committee was formed by the Post-Graduate Education Committee to investigate the problem, set guidelines for possible College programs, and make recommendations for implementation. The Sub-Committee met in Washington in September, 1972. Their task was to develop guidelines for graded exercise testing and exercise prescription for both asymptomatic individuals and individuals with known heart disease, and define behavioral objectives for the four key figures in the administration of graded exercise testing and conditioning programs: the physician, the exercise program director, the exercise specialist, and the exercise test technologist.

Sub-Committee members undertook specific writing assignments and prepared a working document for presentation at a workshop at Aspen, Colorado, in December, 1972. Fifteen laboratories were represented in the 4-day workshop where specific guidelines and behavioral objectives were discussed.

The first draft of the *Guidelines* manuscript was

completed in February, 1973. The Sub-Committee reported on the progress of the *Guidelines* and future plans for implementation at an open meeting during the 1973 Annual Meeting of the College at Seattle. The Sub-Committee having completed its task was disbanded and the manuscript was edited by the Post-Graduate Education Committee. A working document was presented to representatives from 32 laboratories at a second Aspen workshop held in December, 1973. Further revisions were made by appropriate subgroups and the final draft was submitted to the Publications Committee.

The involvement of physicians, physiologists, and physical educators from 32 laboratories located in 19 states and 3 Canadian provinces assured that the *Guidelines* reflected the many different views of graded exercise testing and exercise prescription. The format of the *Guidelines* was initially developed as a descriptive treatment of how to organize and administer graded exercise testing and prescription. No references were included in the text and since so many persons contributed, no individual credits were made. The *Guidelines* included the application of testing and prescription procedures for the entire population. The Behavioral Objectives were the first attempt to develop outlines of the competencies required for the personnel involved in exercise programs. The Behavioral Objectives have assisted with the development of programs to prepare personnel and in the self-evaluation of the professionals in the field.

The first edition of the *Guidelines* enjoyed phenomenal success. Between its publication in May, 1975, and August, 1979, over 18,000 copies were printed and a French Edition was published. During this period interest in physical activity programs for asymptomatic persons and for patients with cardiovascular and respiratory disease became apparent. Concurrent acceptance of the American College of Sports Medicine certification programs for the Exercise Test Technologist, Exercise Specialist, and Exercise Program Director resulted in the College establishing the Standing Committee, Preventive and Rehabilitative Exercise Programs.

These developments and the experience gained with the organization and administration of workshops and certification programs emphasized the need for a revision of the *Guidelines*. The format of the first edition of the *Guidelines* has been maintained but updated in the second edition to reflect the most recent concepts and developments in the field. Many additional members of the College and of other organizations have given substantially of their time and efforts and have made major contributions through comments, written materials, and editorial assistance. The American College of Sports Medicine is indebted to the individuals who have unselfishly contributed directly and indirectly to the development of the second edition of the *Guidelines* and hopes that the *Guidelines* provide a useful document for professionals in the field of graded exercise testing, exercise prescription and rehabilitation of persons with cardiovascular disease.

Contents

List of Tables

1

Guidelines for Evaluation of Participant Health Status Prior to Exercise Testing

Persons of any age may significantly increase their habitual levels of physical activity safely if there are no contraindications to exercise and a rational program is developed. For physically inactive persons there is no assurance that they can exercise safely. There is even less assurance that they will undertake exercise of the appropriate type, duration, intensity, frequency, and progression. Initially, physically inactive persons should be encouraged to participate in a supervised program primarily to learn how to exercise properly. For participants with coronary heart disease (CHD) risk factors or those with known cardiovascular, pulmonary or other diseases in which increased metabolic rates may be harmful, increases in physical activity for the purpose of physical conditioning should be carried out with supervision. The following guidelines are suggested for the evaluation of persons wishing to enter an exercise program or to change the type, intensity, or duration of their physical activity.

A. PRELIMINARY MEDICAL EVALUATION

The age and health status of participants are the major determinants in establishing appropriate screening and supervisory procedures for graded exercise testing and exercise programs. Participant categories based on variables such as age, symptoms, physical activity, CHD risk-factors, and disease have been determined pragmatically after the evaluation of many thousands of presumed asymptomatic individuals and patients with CHD (Table 1).

B. CATEGORIES OF CANDIDATE FOR AN EXERCISE PROGRAM

Category A: Asymptomatic, physically active persons of any age without CHD risk factors or disease will usually require little supervision if the current type, intensity, and duration of physical activity is maintained. They may require counsel and supervision if their exercise program is interrupted by injury, sickness, or the appearance of cardiorespiratory symptoms. Depending on the severity of the problem, reclassification into a different category may be necessary. Assistance may be required for persons wishing to change the type, intensity, or duration of physical activity. An individual's knowledge, functional capacity, age, and the degree of change in activity determines the assistance required. It is advisable for most persons, particularly those 35 years and older, to consult a physician and subsequently discuss changes in their current program with a certified exercise program director or exercise specialist. By definition, *functional capacity* is the value in METS or oxygen

TABLE 1. CLASSIFICATION BY AGE AND HEALTH STATUS OF PARTICIPANTS FOR EXERCISE TESTING

Category

A	Asymptomatic, physically active persons of any age without CHD risk factors or disease.
B	Asymptomatic, physically inactive persons less than 35 years of age without CHD risk factors or disease.
C	Asymptomatic physically inactive persons 35 years and older without CHD risk factors or disease.
D	Asymptomatic physically active or inactive persons of any age with CHD risk factors but no known disease.
E	Asymptomatic persons of any age with known disease.
F	Symptomatic, physically active persons clinically stable for 6 months or longer.
G	Symptomatic, physically inactive persons clinically stable for 6 months or longer.
H	Symptomatic persons with recent onset of CHD or a change in disease status (Example: Recent myocardial infarction, unstable angina, coronary artery bypass surgery).
I	Persons for whom exercise is contraindicated (See Table 3, Contraindications for Exercise and Exercise Testing).

uptake for the highest exercise intensity completed. After a preliminary medical evaluation the functional capacity of persons in Category A may be determined by a field test or graded exercise test. If a graded exercise test is used, administration should be by qualified exercise test personnel. A field test may be self-administered or administered by a person qualified in graded exercise testing. A field test consists of stepping, walking, walking-running, or running for a period of approximately 15 minutes at the highest intensity the participant can maintain. The field test may take place on firm level terrain, a track, a treadmill, a bicycle ergometer, or steps. The functional capacity may be estimated in METS (Appendix F). The exercise prescription may be calculated from a maximum heart rate obtained during the field test. *Maximum heart rate* is defined as the highest heart rate attainable during an all-out effort. The maximum heart rate during a field test may be obtained by ECG or by palpation of the pulse. The latter is obtained during the immediate post-exercise period by counting pulse beats for 10 seconds and multiplying by 6.

Category B: Asymptomatic, physically inactive persons under 35 years of age without CHD risk factors or CHD, who wish to increase their habitual level of physical activity, may do so with minimal risk. If there are questions about health status of individuals who have not had a medical evaluation during the previous year, they should consult with a physician. The exercise prescription may be prepared by using the functional capacity and maximum heart rate obtained through either a field test or a graded exercise test as described for persons in Category A.

Categories C and D: Inactive, asymptomatic persons 35 years of age or older without CHD risk factors or CHD and asymptomatic persons of any age with CHD risk factors (Table 2) but no CHD, should have a complete medical evaluation and a graded exercise

TABLE 2. MAJOR CHD RISK FACTORS AND PREDISPOSING PROBLEMS OF CARDIOVASCULAR DISEASE

CHD Risk Factors:
1. Hypertension
2. Hyperlipidemia
3. Cigarette smoking
4. Electrocardiographic abnormalities
   a. Evidence of old myocardial infarction
   b. Ischemic ST-T changes
   c. Conduction defects
   d. Arrhythmia
   e. Left-ventricular hypertrophy

Predisposing Problems:
1. Family history of coronary heart disease before age 60.
2. Sedentary life style
3. Type A coronary prone behavior pattern with stressful occupation and lifestyle
4. Diabetes mellitus
5. Hyperuricemia
6. Obesity

test. This test may be administered by persons certified in exercise testing with a physician in the testing area. The physician need not be in visual contact with the subject but must know that the graded exercise test is in progress and be responsible for the safety of the participant.

Categories E, F, and G: Asymptomatic persons with known CHD and physically active persons with stable status (healed myocardial infarction, angina pectoris, pulmonary disease, or claudication) and physically inactive persons with clinically stable symptoms need careful evaluation of specific medical problems and required medications. The graded exercise test must be administered by persons certified in graded exercise testing with a physician in visual contact with the patient during the test.

Category H: Symptomatic individuals or persons with recent changes in disease status require the same careful evaluation and testing as those in preceding categories E–G. In addition, a thorough careful assessment is needed of signs and symptoms, ECG, and of the type and dosage of medication.

Category I: Persons for whom exercise is contraindicated should not be admitted to an exercise program until the medical problems have been evaluated and treated. Many Category I patients have problems in which exercise is contraindicated. Others have not had their disease status controlled adequately to allow exercise or even exercise testing to be performed safely (Table 3). Patients in this second group may be treated until improvement of the medical problems allow re-assignment to Category H or G. Abnormal heart rhythms and conduction disturbances may be controlled by a change in medication or the use of a pacemaker. Severe valvular diseases or coronary artery obstruction may be improved by surgery. Pulmonary disease patients may be improved with drugs. These examples indicate some types of cardiac and respiratory problems that may be improved sufficiently to allow exercise to be safe.

Some physicians in private practice find that screening patients prior to increasing habitual exercise is of great value in primary prevention and developing and maintaining patient rapport. Other physicians, because of a lack of facilities or qualified personnel, experience difficulty with exercise screening and exercise prescription. Under these circumstances, a central referral laboratory with qualified technical and medical personnel for exercise testing, prescription, and program supervision may be utilized. The information obtained from evaluation and testing should be sent promptly to the referring physician and others involved with patient care. This is particularly important in Category I patients who may need immediate medical guidance.

In summary, the limited availability of qualified health personnel and facilities in relation to the large volume of medical evaluations and graded exercise testing required to comply with these recommendations necessitates discretion in their implementation. The degree of medical supervision of graded exercise tests proposed varies from situations in which there may be no physician present, the physician is present but not in visual contact, and the physician is in visual contact with the participant. The appropriate protocol is based on the age, health status, and physical activity level of the person to be tested. All tests should be administered by a person qualified in graded exercise testing, preferably persons certified as an exercise test technologist, exercise specialist, or exercise program director and a physician when necessary.

C. MEDICAL EVALUATION

Information to aid in the screening of persons planning to increase physical activity is obtained from a medical evaluation. The medical evaluation should include (Appendix B):

1. *Comprehensive Medical History.* Personal and surgical medical history, family health history, and current life-style health habits (e.g. cigarette smoking, diet, alcohol intake, habitual physical activity, working environment, stresses) should be evaluated. Any history of chest discomfort, pressure, pain or anginal equivalent, arrhythmias, shortness of breath, intermittent claudication, other symptoms and signs related to cardiovascular or pulmonary disease, or orthopedic problems that may limit exercise should be considered.

2. *Physical Examination.* Those participants in categories A and B should have had a physical examination by the referring physician no longer than 1 year prior to the exercise test. Those in categories C–H should have a physical examination immediately prior to the exercise test. Special consideration during the physical examination should be given to the signs and symptoms related to cardiorespiratory disease and other contraindications to exercise testing (Table 3). These include: *(a)* precordial activity such as apical

impulse, extra-cardiac sounds and thrills, murmurs, systolic "clicks", gallop rhythm (S3 and S4), arrhythmias; *(b)* bruits over the carotids, abdomen, and groin; *(c)* carotid, brachial, abdominal, femoral, popliteal, posterior tibial, and dorsalis pedis pulses; *(d)* evidence of pulmonary disease and chest deformity; *(e)* edema, hepatomegaly; *(f)* xanthoma, arcus lipoides, bilateral ear lobe creases; *(g)* bone and joint abnormalities (thumb sign, hyperextensibility).

3. *Laboratory Evaluation.* A record and an interpretation of a twelve-lead resting electrocardiogram (ECG), resting systolic and diastolic blood pressure must accompany the participant's medical history and results of the physical examination. Comprehensive blood counts, screening profile, lipid analysis, cardiac radionuclide study, echocardiogram and coronary arteriography results, chest x ray and pertinent bone x rays may be helpful if available but are not essential. If the patient has pulmonary disease, recent appropriate pulmonary test results should be available.

Data collected during a graded exercise test may be used in diagnosis and prognosis of cardiovascular disease, evaluation of functional capacity, development of an exercise prescription, and determination of the effectiveness of such therapeutic interventions as exercise, drugs, and cardiovascular surgery. Testing methods and other considerations are discussed in Chapter 2.

2

Guidelines for Graded Exercise Test Administration

A. INTRODUCTION

Guidelines for the administration of a graded exercise test are recommendations based on the current state of the art of graded exercise testing and are not designed to be standards of procedure. The guidelines present a rational approach to graded exercise testing on the premise that qualified test personnel have legitimate reasons for making modifications under specific sets of circumstances.

Since the first edition of these guidelines there has been wider recognition of the functional assessment, diagnostic, and prognostic uses of graded exercise testing. Uses include evaluating the functional capacity of asymptomatic persons as well as defining the hazards and opportunities for increased physical activity for persons at risk because of suspected or documented cardiorespiratory diseases. Although the functional capacities of these two categories of test participants may vary greatly, the guidelines for graded exercise test administration are similar. Persons in participant categories A through F may be tested in community or hospital based facilities while patients in participant categories G, H, and I should usually be tested in a hospital based or an equivalent facility with physician support (Table 1).

B. HISTORY, PHYSICAL EXAMINATION, AND CONTRAINDICATIONS

The physicians performing the physical examination prior to graded exercise testing should be familiar with participants' relevant past and present medical history with particular emphasis on cardiovascular events as outlined in Chapter 1.

Medical conditions which require consideration before increasing physical activity, whether during inpatient exercise, a graded exercise test, occupational tasks, or recreational pursuits are outlined in Table 3.

TABLE 3. CONTRAINDICATIONS FOR EXERCISE AND EXERCISE TESTING (Out-of-Hospital Setting)

1. *Contraindications*
    1. Acute myocardial infarction
    2. Unstable or at-rest angina pectoris
    3. Dangerous arrhythmias (ventricular tachycardia or any rhythm significantly compromising cardiac function)
    4. History suggesting excessive medication effects (digitalis, diuretics, psychotropic agents)
    5. Manifest circulatory insufficiency (congestive heart failure)
    6. Severe aortic stenosis

TABLE 3. CONTRAINDICATIONS FOR EXERCISE AND EXERCISE TESTING (Out-of-Hospital Setting)

---

  7. Severe left ventricular outflow tract obstructive disease (IHSS)
  8. Suspected or known dissecting aneurysm
  9. Active or suspected myocarditis or cardiomyopathy (within the past year)
 10. Thrombophlebitis—known or suspected
 11. Recent embolism, systemic or pulmonary
 12. Recent or active infectious episodes (including upper respiratory infections)
 13. High dose of phenothiazine agents
2. *Relative Contraindications**
  1. Uncontrolled or high-rate supraventricular arrhythmias
  2. Repetitive or frequent ventricular ectopic activity
  3. Untreated severe systemic or pulmonary hypertension
  4. Ventricular aneurysm
  5. Moderate aortic stenosis
  6. Severe myocardial obstructive syndromes (subvalvular, muscular or membranous obstructions)
  7. Marked cardiac enlargement
  8. Uncontrolled metabolic disease (diabetes, thyrotoxicosis, myxedema)
  9. Toxemia or complications of pregnancy
3. *Condition Requiring Special Consideration and/or Precautions*
  1. Conduction disturbances
     a. Complete atrioventricular block
     b. Left bundle branch block
     c. Wolff-Parkinson-White anomaly or syndrome
     d. Lown-Ganong-Levine syndrome
     e. Bifascicular block (with or without 1st° block)

TABLE 3.   CONTRAINDICATIONS FOR EXERCISE AND
EXERCISE TESTING (Out-of-Hospital Setting)

---

 2. Controlled arrhythmias
 3. Fixed rate pacemaker
 4. Mitral valve prolapse (click-murmur) syndrome
 5. Angina pectoris and other manifestations of coronary insufficiency
 6. Certain medications
  a. Digitalis, diuretics, psychotropic drugs
  b. Beta-blocking and drugs of related action
  c. Nitrates
  d. Antihypertensive drugs
 7. Electrolyte disturbance
 8. Clinically severe hypertension (diastolic above 110, grade III retinopathy)
 9. Cyanotic heart disease
10. Intermittent or fixed right-to-left shunt
11. Severe anemia (hemoglobin below 10 gm/dl
12. Marked obesity (20% above optimal body weight)
13. Renal, hepatic, and other metabolic insufficiency
14. Overt psychoneurotic disturbances requiring therapy
15. Neuromuscular, musculoskeletal, orthopedic, or arthritic disorders which would prevent activity
16. Moderate to severe pulmonary disease
17. Intermittent claudication
18. Diabetes

---

*In the practice of medicine the benefits of evaluation often exceed the risks for patients with these relative contraindications.

The medical evaluation outlined in Chapter 1 should determine if any of these contraindications for exercise exist. If participants are taking medications, a decision whether or not to continue the medications is required prior to the exercise test. If the primary purpose of the graded exercise test is to establish the participant's functional capacity, then the regular medication schedule should be continued. In no case should a drug be discontinued without explicit consent of the referring physician.

C. SIGNED INFORMED CONSENT

Prior to administration of the graded exercise test, the participant must receive an explanation of the test procedures from a qualified staff member. This explanation must include a description of the possible risks and discomforts and the potential benefits to be expected. Following the explanation, the participant, legal guardian, or both must be asked if there are any questions that have not been answered. The participant or legal guardian and the individual responsible for administering the test must sign the informed consent document (Appendix A). Before the patient begins the graded exercise test, a qualified person should briefly demonstrate the test procedure.

D. TEST PROTOCOL

The exercise test should be graded according to energy requirements in METS. One *MET* is the equivalent of a resting oxygen consumption taken in a sitting

TABLE 4.   ENERGY REQUIREMENTS IN METS FOR HORIZONTAL AND UPHILL JOGGING/RUNNING*

a. Outdoors on solid surface

% Grade	mph	5	6	7	7.5	8	9	10
	m/min	134	161	188	201	215	241	268
0		8.6	10.2	11.7	12.5	13.3	14.8	16.3
2.5		10.3	12.3	14.1	15.1	16.1	17.9	19.7
5.0		12.0	14.3	16.5	17.7	18.8	21.0	23.2
7.5		13.8	16.4	18.9	20.2	21.6	24.1	26.6
10.0		15.5	18.5	21.4	22.8	24.3	27.2	
12.5		17.2	20.6	23.8	25.4	27.1		

b. On the treadmill

| % Grade | mph | 5 | 6 | 7 | 7.5 | 8 | 9 | 10 |
	m/min	134	161	188	201	215	241	268
0		8.6	10.2	11.7	12.5	13.3	14.8	16.3
2.5		9.5	11.2	12.9	13.8	14.7	16.3	18.0
5.0		10.3	12.3	14.1	15.1	16.1	17.9	19.7
7.5		11.2	13.3	15.3	16.4	17.4	19.4	21.4
10.0		12.0	14.3	16.5	17.7	18.8	21.0	23.2
12.5		12.9	15.4	17.7	19.0	20.2	22.5	24.9
15.0		13.8	16.4	18.9	20.3	21.6	24.1	26.6

*Differences in energy expenditures are accounted for by the effects of wind resistance.

TABLE 5. ENERGY EXPENDITURE IN METS DURING BICYCLE ERGOMETRY

| Body Weight | | Exercise Rate (kgm/min and Watts) | | | | | | | |
kg	lbs	300 / 50	450 / 75	600 / 100	750 / 125	900 / 150	1050 / 175	1200 / 200	(kgm/min) (Watts)
50	110	5.1	6.9	8.6	10.3	12.0	13.7	15.4	
60	132	4.3	5.7	7.1	8.6	10.0	11.4	12.9	
70	154	3.7	4.9	6.1	7.3	8.6	9.8	11.0	
80	176	3.2	4.3	5.4	6.4	7.5	8.6	9.6	
90	198	2.9	3.8	4.8	5.7	6.7	7.6	8.6	
100	220	2.6	3.4	4.3	5.1	6.0	6.9	7.7	

NOTE: $\dot{V}O_2$ for zero load pedaling is approximately 550 ml/min for 70 to 80 kg subjects.

TABLE 6. APPROXIMATE ENERGY REQUIREMENTS IN METS FOR HORIZONTAL AND GRADE WALKING

% Grade	mph	1.7	2.0	2.5	3.0	3.4	3.75
	m/min	*45.6*	*53.7*	*67.0*	*80.5*	*91.2*	*100.5*
0		2.3	2.5	2.9	3.3	3.6	3.9
2.5		2.9	3.2	3.8	4.3	4.8	5.2
5.0		3.5	3.9	4.6	5.4	5.9	6.5
7.5		4.1	4.6	5.5	6.4	7.1	7.8
10.0		4.6	5.3	6.3	7.4	8.3	9.1
12.5		5.2	6.0	7.2	8.5	9.5	10.4
15.0		5.8	6.6	8.1	9.5	10.6	11.7
17.5		6.4	7.3	8.9	10.5	11.8	12.9
20.0		7.0	8.0	9.8	11.6	13.0	14.2
22.5		7.6	8.7	10.6	12.6	14.2	15.5
25.0		8.2	9.4	11.5	13.6	15.3	16.8

position: approximately 3.5 ml/kg•min or 1.0 kcal/kg•hr. METS during exercise are determined by dividing metabolic rate during exercise by the metabolic rate at rest. The MET cost of treadmill exercise is independent of body weight (Table 4), but the MET cost of bicycle ergometry is dependent on body weight (Table 5). METS may be estimated from the exercise intensity performed (Tables 4 to 7 and Appendix E) or by calculating oxygen uptake from measurements of minute ventilation and expired gas composition. Either method may be used effectively in exercise testing and prescription.

TABLE 7.   ENERGY EXPENDITURE IN METS DURING STEPPING AT DIFFERENT RATES ON STEPS OF DIFFERENT HEIGHTS

Step Height		Steps/min			
cm	in	12	18	24	30
0	0	1.2	1.8	2.4	3.0
4	1.6	1.5	2.3	3.1	3.8
8	3.2	1.9	2.8	3.7	4.6
12	4.7	2.2	3.3	4.4	5.5
16	6.3	2.5	3.8	5.0	6.3
20	7.9	2.8	4.3	5.7	7.1
24	9.4	3.2	4.8	6.3	7.9
28	11.0	3.5	5.2	7.0	8.7
32	12.6	3.8	5.7	7.7	9.6
36	14.2	4.1	6.2	8.3	10.4
40	15.8	4.5	6.7	9.0	11.2

E. ELECTROCARDIOGRAM (ECG)

Immediately prior to the graded exercise test a standard 12 lead ECG should be recorded on a participant in a supine position. The purpose of this ECG is to detect contraindications to exercise testing and provide a baseline for comparing similar tracings taken during recovery. Additional pre-exercise ECG tracings should be taken with the participant's posture equivalent to that used during exercise. If ECG tracings are taken during hyperventilation, participants should be in a posture similar to that used during the graded exercise test.

Some laboratories record the ECG during the 30 to 60 seconds of hyperventilation prior to the graded exercise test to determine if ischemic type ECG changes will occur. Occasionally this procedure will produce changes similar to "ischemic patterns" seen with exercise in certain conditions, i.e. "vasoregulatory asthenia" and the mitral valve prolapse "click-murmur" syndrome. Such hyperventilation responses do not preclude significant coronary obstructive disease but their appearance suggests the increased probability of a "false positive" exercise test. "False positive" exercise tests suggesting "ischemia" in the absence of significant ischemic heart disease have been observed more frequently in women than in men. Exact indications for having patients perform hyperventilation and the significance of a positive exercise test in women has not been established and clinical judgment is required.

During the graded exercise test a minimum of precordial lead in the V_5 position must be recorded.

Sensitivity and specificity can be improved by using additional leads. When multichannel ECG monitoring systems are available minimal recordings of the following three leads are recommended:

(a) An anterior precordial lead in the V_1 or V_2 position
(b) A "lateral" or "apical" precordial lead in the V_5 position
(c) An inferior lead such as AVF or its equivalent

The ECG should be continuously monitored by oscilloscope and recordings taken at the end of each minute of exercise and when significant ECG changes are noted. The ECG monitoring and intermittent recordings should be continued throughout the post-exercise recovery period. Before the participant is released a 12 lead ECG recording should be made to document that the ECG configuration has returned to the pre-exercise condition.

Certain medications are known to alter the ECG responses to exercise (pulse rate, ST segments, T waves, and QT interval). If in use, these medications should be considered when interpretation of the exercise ECG is made. "False positive" tests suggesting "ischemia" may occur in the absence of significant ischemic heart disease when ST–T wave changes result from ingested digitalis preparations or diuretics which have induced hypokalemia. "False negative" interpretations, where ST–T changes are masked, are alleged to result from treatment with drugs such as propranolol, quinidine, or reserpine. Details of these changes may be found in Appendix D.

F. BLOOD PRESSURE

Arterial blood pressure measured by the auscultatory method should be determined at rest, during exercise, immediately following exercise, and during recovery using a high quality stethoscope and mercury manometer. The pre-exercise pressure should be recorded with the subject in the posture to be used during the graded exercise test. During exercise, blood pressure is generally recorded during the last half minute of each exercise intensity or every other exercise intensity if the duration of each is 1 minute. Arterial blood pressures should be periodically monitored during recovery until they return to near pre-exercise levels.

G. TERMINATION OF EXERCISE TEST

Graded exercise tests conducted by non-physicians should be stopped for the reasons listed. Physicians conducting graded exercise tests may use other criteria according to clinical considerations as with patients in category H. The signs and symptoms of exercise intolerance presented are a guide to assist in a decision to terminate a graded exercise test.

1. Maximum oxygen uptake. The most definitive criterion for the termination of the graded exercise test is the attainment of maximum oxygen uptake ($\dot{V}O_2$ max), "true maximum capacity." *Maximum oxygen uptake* is attained when, with further increments in the intensity of exercise, $\dot{V}O_2$ does not increase. Physically conditioned

persons can consistently reach a $\dot{V}O_2$ max but sedentary persons and symptomatic persons reach $\dot{V}O_2$ max with difficulty or are unable to reach it. If the graded exercise test is stopped by the physician or certified professional staff because of the appearance of participant discomfort or other criteria for exercise termination, $\dot{V}O_2$ max most likely will not be attained. Even at the point of exercise limiting fatigue, most poorly conditioned persons will not display a plateau of $\dot{V}O_2$. In spite of this, an endpoint in graded exercise determined by signs and symptoms, ECG changes, blood pressure, heart rate, and respiratory responses is useful as an evaluative technique and to determine the exercise prescription. This is the maximum level of exercise achieved by the participant and may be estimated in METS and referred to as functional capacity.

2. Signs and symptoms of exertional intolerance.
    a. Dizziness or near syncope
    b. Angina, regardless of the presence or absence of ECG abnormalities consistent with myocardial ischemia. (Subjective angina ratings of the +3 level may be used if the exercising participant has been evaluated previously by a physician and the reliability of the subjective ratings has been established.)*
    c. Nausea
    d. Marked dyspnea
    e. Unusual or severe fatigue

---

*NOTE: +3 angina = moderate discomfort, +1 = definite unquestionable discomfort, +2 = mild, +4 = equivalent to most severe discomfort ever experienced.

  f. Severe claudication or other pain

  g. Staggering or persistent unsteadiness

  h. Mental confusion

  i. Facial expression signifying severe distress

  j. Loss of sustained vigor of palpable pulse

  k. Cyanosis or severe pallor

  l. Lack of rapid erythematous return of skin color after brief firm compression

 3. Electrocardiographic changes

  a. ST–T segment horizontal or "divergent" displacement of 0.2 mV above or below the resting isoelectric line for at least 0.08 second duration after the junction ("J") point.

  b. Ventricular arrhythmia

   (1) Ventricular tachycardia (three or more successive ectopic ventricular complexes)

   (2) Continuous bigeminal or trigeminal ectopic ventricular complexes

   (3) Frequent unifocal or multifocal ectopic ventricular complexes amounting to greater than 30% (trigeminy) of the total beats per minute

   (4) Due to the difficulty in differentiating between supraventricular and ventricular rhythms, unless well interpreted, supraventricular atrial complexes with aberrant ventricular conduction should be interpreted in the same way as ectopic ventricular beats

  c. Atrial-ventricular or ventricular conduction disturbances

   (1) Second degree AV Block, Mobitz Type I (Wenckebach)

      (2) Second degree AV Block, Mobitz Type II
      (3) Third degree (complete) AV Block
      (4) Sudden Left Bundle Branch Block

4. Blood pressure responses. If systolic blood pressure (SBP) fails to rise with increasing exercise intensities (except as a result of familiarization in the early stages) or if SBP shows a drop of 10 mm Hg or more, termination of the exercise test is usually indicated. An increase in SBP to the range of 250 mm Hg or above is considered by some authorities as an indication for stopping exercise but there is a lack of published reports indicating complications associated with high SBP during exercise. A diastolic rise of more than 20 mm Hg or a rise above 110 to 120 mm Hg is often considered an indication that the test should be terminated.

5. Heart rate responses. Exercise heart rate will vary according to age, anxiety, disease, medications, and functional capacity. Maximal heart rates for apparently healthy individuals 15 years and over may be estimated either by subtracting the participant's age from 220 (low estimate) or one half their age from 210 (high estimate). Although these estimates may be used as a guide in test termination, they should not be used as predetermined termination points. It is important to remember that even for asymptomatic adults the range of maximal heart rates for any one age is quite large (standard deviation: ± ten beats per minute) and that patients may have much lower maximal rates. Symptom and sign limited tests

are likely to be more useful. Once the maximal heart rate has been determined experimentally by a graded exercise test, it may usually be used effectively in exercise prescription.

6. Respiratory responses. Marked dyspnea or cyanosis may be observed when individuals with pulmonary impairment exercise. Termination of the exercise test is recommended when the above symptoms or signs are observed.

7. Malfunctioning equipment. In the event that there is an equipment malfunction or the ECG monitoring system fails to give an interpretable ECG, the test should be terminated and the problem corrected before proceeding with the graded exercise test.

H.   POST-EXERCISE TEST

During the early part of the recovery period the participant should be in a supine resting position or should exercise at low intensity (zero load 50 to 60 RPM on the bicycle ergometer; 2 mph, 0% grade on the treadmill; stepping forward and backward on level at 25 steps per minute). The participant *should not be kept motionless* (for more than 10 seconds) in the standing position or in the seated position with the legs down. The ECG and blood pressure should be periodically recorded during at least eight minutes of recovery or, if abnormal, until they return to near the pre-exercise conditions.

I. EMERGENCY PROCEDURES

1. All personnel concerned with an exercise program should be trained in cardiopulmonary resuscitation (CPR) at the basic rescue level.
2. The exercise program director or laboratory supervisor when possible should be trained in Advanced Cardiac Life Support.
3. Emergency equipment and drugs (Table 8) must be available in the immediate areas or through a mobile emergency unit and telephone call system.
4. Telephone numbers for emergency assistance should be clearly posted at all telephones.
5. Evacuation plans should be established and posted. Every staff person should be thoroughly familiar with all specific duties and evacuation procedures required in an emergency.
6. Procedures (code team drills) should be practiced on a regularly scheduled basis (Table 9).

Suggested reading materials for all staff personnel:

1. Standards for Cardiopulmonary Resuscitation (CPR) and Emergency Cardiac Care (ECC). Supplement to the *JAMA; (227),* 833–868; February 18, 1974. Revised *JAMA; (244),* 453–509; August 1, 1980.
2. Advanced Cardiac Life Support Manual: The American Heart Association, 1975.

TABLE 8.   EMERGENCY EQUIPMENT AND DRUGS

1. Defibrillator—monitor with ECG electrodes—defibrillator paddles or portable DC defibrillator and portable ECG monitor
2. Airways—nasopharyngeal and oral (endotracheal desirable)
3. Face mask and Robert Shaw valve
4. Oxygen
5. Suction apparatus
6. Syringes and needles
7. Intravenous sets
8. Intravenous stand
9. Adhesive tape
10. Laryngoscope (desirable)

1. Sodium bicarbonate I.V.
2. Catecholamine agents
   Epinephrine I.V.
   Isoproterenol I.V.
   Dobutamine I.V.
3. Atropine sulfate
4. Antiarrhythmic agents
   Lidocaine I.V.
   Procainamide I.V.
   Propranolol I.V./oral
5. Morphine sulfate
6. Calcium chloride
7. Vasoactive agent
   Norepinephrine
8. Corticosteroids
   Methylprednisolone sodium succinate
   Dexamethasone phosphate
9. Digoxin I.V./oral
10. Lasix I.V.
11. Dextrose 5% in water
12. Nitroglycerin tablets
13. Amyl nitrite pearls

NOTE: Although these items of equipment and drugs are suggested for emergency use where possible, it may be more advisable to be organized into a hospital emergency call system. (Also see reference 1 above).

TABLE 9.   EXERCISE RELATED CARDIOVASCULAR EMERGENCIES

Basic Causes	Signs and Symptoms	Emergency Procedures
I. CARDIAC ARREST		
A. Ventricular Fibrillation	See Standards for CPR and ECC Supplement to JAMA (227), 833–868, February 18, 1974. Revised JAMA; (244): 453–509: August 1, 1980.	Defibrillate
B. Cardiac Standstill (Ventricular Asystole)		Defibrillate
II. LOW CARDIAC OUTPUT STATES		
A. Inadequate Venous Return	Tachycardia, Low B.P., Pallor, Dizziness	Supine with legs elevated Isometric or low level dynamic exercise I.V. and/or oral fluid vasopressor medication

B. Arrhythmias
  1. Tachycardia
 	
  2. Bradycardia
  3. Premature ventricular and atrial contractions
	Must define by ECG	Stop exercise, supine position
		Watch B.P. closely
		I.V. medications
		D.C. countershock or defibrillation as indicated
		Treat for inadequate venous return (i.e. Atropine, Isuprel) or specific treatment depending on ECG diagnosis

C. Myocardial Failure	Inordinate Dyspnea, Rales, Gallop Rhythm	Stop exercise, sitting position
		Oxygen administration
		Positive pressure breathing
		Drugs
		  1. Use of sublingual nitroglycerin should be considered
		  2. Morphine

D. Drug Induced Low Output
  1. Beta Blockers
  2. Diuretics
  3. Antihypertensives
	Slow Heart Rate
	Low Blood Pressure
		Supine with legs elevated
		I.V. fluids if appropriate
		Drugs appropriate to counteract cause

TABLE 9. EXERCISE RELATED CARDIOVASCULAR EMERGENCIES

III. ISCHEMIC STATUS

A. Chest Pain, Unrelent- ing	ECG Evidence of Ischemia	Stop exercise, immediate O_2, nitroglycerin, possible Inde- ral, possible hospitalization
B. Myocardial Infarct	ECG Evidence of Infarct, Ischemia or Supporting Clinical Evidence	Hospitalize, treat arrhythmia and circulatory inadequacy
C. Papillary Muscle Dysfunction	Loud Systolic Murmur	Sitting position Nitroglycerin Hospitalization if it persists
D. Cerebral	Ataxia, Dizziness, Impaired Consciousness	Stop exercise, supine rest, monitor B.P., I.V. fluids
E. Gastrointestinal	Nausea, Vomiting, Vasovagal Syncope	Stop exercise, supine rest, emesis basin

NOTE: Cardiovascular Collapse. A general term applied to impairment of the cardiovascular system of such severity that the subject cannot stand or walk. This table does not include those symptoms/signs which may occur during exercise testing which result in cardiovascular collapse.

3

Guidelines for Exercise Prescription

Exercise prescription includes the type, intensity, duration, frequency, and progression of physical activity. These five components are applicable to the development of exercise programs for persons regardless of age, functional capacity, and presence or absence of CHD risk factors or CHD. The maximum safe exercise prescription for any individual is best determined from measurements of heart rate, ECG, arterial blood pressure, and functional capacity obtained during the graded exercise test.

Based on the existing evidence concerning exercise prescription for asymptomatic adults, the American College of Sports Medicine has made the following recommendations for the quantity and quality of exercise for developing and maintaining cardiorespiratory fitness and body composition.

1. Type of activity: Any activity that uses large muscle groups, that can be maintained continuously, and is rhythmical and aerobic in nature, e.g. running-jogging, walking-hiking, swimming, skating, bicycling, rowing, cross-country skiing, rope skipping, and various endurance game activities.

2. Intensity of conditioning: 60 to 90% of maximum heart rate or 50 to 85% of $\dot{V}O_2$ max.
3. Duration of conditioning: 15 to 60 minutes of continuous or discontinuous aerobic activity. Duration is dependent on the intensity of the activity, thus lower intensity activity should be conducted over a longer period of time. Endurance conditioning is more readily attained in longer duration programs. Lower to moderate intensity activity of longer duration is recommended for non-athletic adults because of potential hazards and compliance problems associated with high intensity activity.
4. Frequency of conditioning: 3 to 5 days per week.
5. Rate of progression: In most cases, the conditioning effect allows individuals to increase the total work done per session. In continuous exercise this occurs by an increase in intensity, duration, or some combination of the two. The possibilities for increasing total work are more numerous in discontinuous exercise because of the different opportunities for increasing the average intensity. The most significant conditioning effects may be observed during the first 6 to 8 weeks of the exercise program. The physician, exercise program director, or exercise specialist must adjust the exercise prescription as these conditioning effects occur depending on the participant category (Table 1), periodic new graded exercise test or merely on the exercise performance during exercise sessions.

The principles of exercise prescription are the same for the asymptomatic and the symptomatic participant.

What will differ is the manner in which the principles are applied, i.e., higher intensity vs. lower intensity, longer duration vs. short duration and daily exercise vs. 3 times per week frequency.

Each exercise session includes a warm-up, 5 to 10 minutes; endurance (aerobic) activity, 15 to 60 minutes; and, cool-down, 5 to 10 minutes. The warm-up period is designed to gradually increase the metabolic rate from the resting level of one MET to the MET level required for conditioning. The warm-up period usually lasts 5 to 10 minutes and includes stretching exercises (joint-readiness), calisthenics or other types of muscle conditioning exercises, and walking or slow jogging. The duration and intensity of each of these activities will depend on environmental conditions, functional capacity, symptomatology, and exercise preference of the participant. For participants who require or prefer greater amounts of muscle strength or endurance, additional calisthenics and exercises utilizing weights may be included (10 to 20 minutes). However, moderate to heavy lifting activities or exercising with weights are not recommended for persons with hypertension, arrhythmias, or poor cardiac reserve. The endurance or aerobic phase of conditioning can be designed to be continuous or discontinuous. It includes aerobic-type activities involving large muscle groups to produce heart rates of prescribed intensity. The cool-down period includes exercises of diminishing intensities, e.g. slower walking or jogging, stretching, and in some cases, relaxation activities.

For asymptomatic, physically active young people modifications in intensity and duration of exercise are a simple matter involving minimal personal risk. Modifying exercise prescription is more difficult for sedentary, older, or symptomatic participants. The degree of risk involved in exercise is a function of the interaction of: (1) the severity of the exercise relative to the habitual intensity of exercise performed, (2) age, (3) functional capacity, (4) health status, (5) risk factors, and (6) symptomatology.

A. TYPE OF EXERCISE

The selection of activities is made on the basis of the individual's functional capacity, physical activity interests, availability of time, equipment and facilities, and the objectives of the exercise program. Physical activities may be conveniently classified in terms of their contribution to the conditioning objectives: (1) cardiorespiratory endurance, (2) flexibility, coordination, and relaxation, (3) muscular strength and endurance.

1. *Cardiorespiratory Endurance Activities.* The intent of exercise prescription is to increase or maintain the functional capacity. To accomplish this goal a portion of each exercise session is devoted to aerobic endurance activities.

Endurance activities may be classified into two groups: (1) physical activities during which the exercise intensity is easily sustained with little variability in heart rate response (e.g. walking, jogging, running, swimming, cycling, cross-country skiing, and skating), and (2) physical activities during which the continuous exercise intensity is not maintained (e.g. dancing, figure skating, mountain hiking, and a variety of games and sports).

When precise control of exercise intensity is necessary, as in the early stages of a conditioning or rehabilitation program, Group 1 activities are recommended. Individual skill levels and personal preference will determine whether Group 1 activities will be performed in a continuous or discontinuous (interval conditioning) exercise format. These activities continue to be useful at all stages of a conditioning program because they enable the participant to expend the most energy per unit of time. Group 2 activities can be extremely useful because of the enjoyment they provide in a physically active setting and their ability to direct the participant's attention away from anxieties, worries, and boredom.

Competitive aspects of games should be supervised to minimize the risk to participants. Modification of game rules is recommended. Such activities should not be included until participants obtain a minimum of exercise intensity of 5 METS and the exercise specialist becomes familiar with the physiologic and psychologic responses of the participants. Without modifications competitive activities are not recommended for the sedentary or multiple risk individuals (participant categories C–H Table 1). For asymptomatic sedentary participants (participant categories C, D, E) a 6 to 10 week conditioning period will usually prepare a participant for game activities. In addition to the graded exercise test, participants in participant categories E–H should have radio telemetry or ambulatory (Holter) ECG monitoring under actual exercise conditions before being released into self-regulated or recreational games.

2. *Flexibility and Relaxation Activities.* Flexibility

exercises can assist with extending and maintaining the range of movement of a joint or a series of joints. Flexibility exercises should be performed slowly with a gradual progression to greater ranges of motion. Dynamic and static movements may be combined by following a slow ballistic movement with a momentarily held static stretch. Although maintenance of flexibility in all joints is important, the lower back is particularly susceptible to chronic soreness and pain. Low back problems may be alleviated by strengthening the abdominal muscles, improving posture, and stretching the lower back and the posterior thigh muscles. Muscle cramping and other musculoskeletal injuries associated with an exercise program predominated by jogging and running, may be avoided by including special stretching exercises for the posterior thigh and lower leg muscles. Exercise can also be designed to relieve neuromuscular tension. Flexibility and relaxation exercises are effective activities during the warm-up and cool-down periods (Chap. 4).

3. *Muscular Strength and Endurance Activities.* These activities have little direct effect on the cardiorespiratory system or the functional capacity. However, many leisure and occupational tasks require arm exercises, e.g. moving, lifting, or holding a weight. The physiologic stress induced by lifting or holding a given weight is proportional to the percentage of maximum strength involved. The maintenance or enhancement of muscle strength and muscle endurance will enable the individual to perform such tasks with less stress.

Muscular strength is acquired by dynamic high-tension low-repetition exercises or through static contractions. Both dynamic lifting procedures and static contractions result in an increased systemic arterial blood pressure. An increased blood pressure increases the work of the heart and its requirements for oxygen. Such lifts may cause a reduction in venous return and result in decreased blood flow to the heart and brain (e.g. Valsalva maneuver). Maximal tension exercises should be discouraged for sedentary symptomatic or multiple risk individuals (participant categories D–H Table 1). Instead, dynamic low-weight exercises should be incorporated into the program for improvement of both muscle strength and endurance. If such activities are used, participants should be trained to make all strength movements while breathing freely without breath-holding. Exhalation on effort should be encouraged. In addition, special attention must be directed toward sufficient warm-up and cool-down, correct structural and functional body position for lifting, and rhythmic performance of the necessary movements. With progress in conditioning most participants will be able to perform safely such tasks as carrying groceries, mowing the lawn, and raking leaves.

B. INTENSITY OF EXERCISE

The most difficult problem in designing exercise programs is the prescription of the appropriate exercise intensity. This requires an individualized exercise prescription and adequate monitoring to ensure that the maximum prescribed intensity is not exceeded. The intensity of exercise may be best expressed as a percentage of functional capacity. The percentage of functional capacity a given individual is able to sustain for a specified conditioning period is quite variable. Marathon runners are able to maintain 80% of functional capacity from 2 to 4 hours, but poorly conditioned individuals exercising at 80% would be fatigued in less than 30 minutes. Such differences in the ability of persons to sustain a given exercise intensity must be taken into consideration in developing the exercise prescription.

Exercise prescription intensities during conditioning sessions should not exceed 90% of the functional capacity nor usually be lower than 60%. The average conditioning intensity for asymptomatic adults is between 70 and 80%. Participants, including cardiac patients, who have a low functional capacity, may initiate their conditioning at 40 to 60% of their functional capacity. Duration can then be set empirically, based on the participant feeling rested and not fatigued within an hour following exercise. The intensity of the exercise may be prescribed by METS or by heart rate.

1. *Exercise Prescription by METS.* Once the participant's health status and functional capacity are known, the exercise intensity can be defined. In general, the results from the graded exercise test are used to establish upper limits of the conditioning intensity. Different considerations may be used for the cardiac patients, depending on the status of their recovery.

The peak and average intensity of exercise may be estimated by determining 90 and 70% of the individual's functional capacity. For a person with a maximum functional capacity of 8 METS:

Peak Conditioning Intensity = .90 × 8 = 7.2 METS

Average Conditioning
Intensity $= .70 \times 8 = 5.6$ METS

There is an alternative method that sets a sliding scale for estimating the average conditioning intensity. The sliding scale allows for the variability due to known differences in the intensity that can be tolerated by persons with different functional capacities. The baseline intensity is set at 60% of the functional capacity in METS. Thus, for persons with functional capacities ranging from 3 to 20 METS:

Functional Capacity (METS)	Percentage Plus Functional Capacity	Average Conditioning Intensity (METS)
3	60 + 3 = 63	(.63 × 3 =) 1.90
5	60 + 5 = 65	3.25
10	60 + 10 = 70	7.00
15	60 + 15 = 75	11.25
20	60 + 20 = 80	16.00

The average exercise intensity during a given conditioning session may be obtained by alternating periods of exercise at higher and lower intensities. If, for example, an exercise intensity of 5.5 METS is prescribed, equal time intervals at 4 and 7 METS will result in the prescribed 5.5 MET average. Thus, any modification can be prescribed precisely. Since the high intensity period is more likely to be hazardous, this format should be approached with caution. As a rule the initial exercise prescription should set exercise intensity about 1 MET lower than estimated until the participant has become accustomed to exercise and the exercise specialist is familiar with the participant response.

For physical activities such as walking, jogging, running, bicycle ergometer exercise, and stepping or stair climbing, the exercise intensity in METS is directly related to the speed of movement, measurable resistance, or mass lifted. Even in these activities the maintenance of the prescribed safe conditioning intensity can be complicated by changes in the environment. Critical environmental factors include: wind, hills, sand, snow, obstacles such as ditches, fences or underbrush, heat or cold, humidity, altitude, pollution, bulky clothing or clothing that obstructs movement, and the weight and size of equipment such as back packs, skis, suitcases, or grocery bags. The problem of exercising at a prescribed conditioning intensity in any activity under most environmental conditions may be solved by using heart rate as an indicator of exercise intensity.

Prescription and maintenance of safe exercise intensities are more difficult in complex individual sports of swimming, skiing, rowing, dual sports such as tennis, handball, or squash, and team sports such as volleyball, softball, soccer, or touch football (Table 10).

TABLE 10.   LEISURE ACTIVITIES IN METS: SPORTS, EXERCISE CLASSES, GAMES, DANCING

	Mean	*Range*
Archery	3.9	3–4
Back Packing	—	5–11
Badminton	5.8	4–9+

TABLE 10. LEISURE ACTIVITIES IN METS: SPORTS, EXERCISE CLASSES, GAMES, DANCING

	Mean	*Range*
Basketball		
Gameplay	8.3	7–12+
Non-game	—	3–9
Billiards	2.5	–
Bowling	—	2–4
Boxing		
In-ring	13.3	–
Sparring	8.3	–
Canoeing, Rowing		
and Kayaking	—	3–8
Conditioning Exercise	—	3–8+
Climbing Hills	7.2	5–10+
Cricket	5.2	4.6–7.4
Croquet	3.5	–
Cycling		
Pleasure or to work	—	3–8+
10 mph	7.0	–
Dancing (Social, Square, Tap)	—	3.7–7.4
Dancing(Aerobic)	—	6–9
Fencing	—	6–10+
Field Hockey	8.0	–
Fishing		
from bank	3.7	2–4
wading in stream	—	5–6
Football (Touch)	7.9	6–10
Golf		
Power cart	—	2–3
Walking (carrying bag or		
pulling cart)	5.1	4–7
Handball	—	8–12+
Hiking (Cross-country)	—	3–7

TABLE 10.   LEISURE ACTIVITIES IN METS: SPORTS,
EXERCISE CLASSES, GAMES, DANCING

	Mean	*Range*
Horseback Riding		
Galloping	8.2	–
Trotting	6.6	–
Walking	2.4	–
Horseshoe Pitching	—	2–3
Hunting (Bow or Gun)		
Small game (walking, carrying light load)	—	3–7
Big game (dragging carcass, walking)	—	3–14
Judo	13.5	–
Mountain Climbing	—	5–10+
Music Playing	—	2–3
Paddleball, Racquetball	9	8–12
Rope Jumping	11	–
60–80 skips/min	9	–
120–140 skips/min	—	11–12
Running		
12 min per mile	8.7	–
11 min per mile	9.4	–
10 min per mile	10.2	–
9 min per mile	11.2	–
8 min per mile	12.5	–
7 min per mile	14.1	–
6 min per mile	16.3	–
Sailing	—	2–5
Scubadiving	—	5–10
Shuffleboard	—	2–3
Skating, Ice and Roller	—	5–8
Skiing, Snow		
Downhill	—	5–8
Cross country	—	6–12+

TABLE 10. LEISURE ACTIVITIES IN METS: SPORTS, EXERCISE CLASSES, GAMES, DANCING

	Mean	*Range*
Skiing, Water	—	5–7
Sledding, Tobogganing	—	4–8
Snowshoeing	9.9	7–14
Squash	—	8–12+
Soccer	—	5–12+
Stairclimbing	—	4–8
Swimming	—	4–8+
Table Tennis	4.1	3–5
Tennis	6.5	4–9+
Volleyball	—	3–6

NOTE: Since 1 MET = 1 kcal/kg•hr multiply the MET value by body wt. of the subject in kg and divide by 60 min per hr to obtain energy expediture in kcal/min.

EXAMPLE:

5 METS = 5 kcal/kg•hr

$$5 \text{ kcal/kg•hr} \times \frac{65 \text{ kg}}{60 \text{ min per hr}} = 5.4 \text{ kcal/min}$$

2. *Exercise Prescription by Heart Rate.* In general, unless disturbed by environmental conditions, psychologic stimuli or disease, a linear relationship exists between heart rate (HR) and exercise intensity. Individual differences will be detected during the graded exercise test. The first method for calculating target heart rate is to plot the slope of the line between the individual's exercise heart rates and the exercise intensity in either METS or $\dot{V}O_2$ (Fig. 1). The

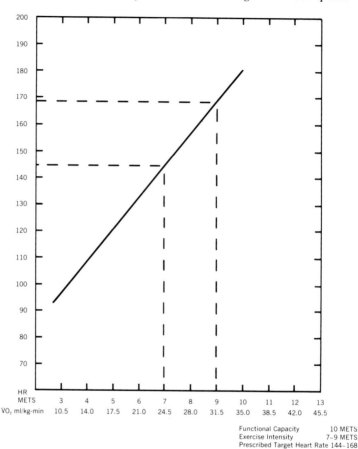

Functional Capacity			10 METS
Exercise Intensity			7–9 METS
Prescribed Target Heart Rate 144–168			

Fig. 1. Plotting the target heart rate.

"maximum" heart rate is the heart rate measured at the highest exercise intensity attained. From this relationship, the heart rate pertaining to a given percent of functional capacity can be obtained. This heart rate value, called the "target" heart rate, may be used for estimating intensity during conditioning.

A second method is to determine the target heart rate for a participant by multiplying the difference between the maximum and resting heart rates by the same percentage that was used to determine the exercise prescription in METS. This value is then added to the resting heart rate to obtain the target heart rate.

For Example:

Maximum Heart Rates (beats per minute)	= 180
Resting Heart Rate	−60
	120
Conditioning Intensity	×70%
	84
Resting Heart Rate	+60
Minimum Training Heart Rate	144

A third method for determining target heart rate is to calculate a given percentage of the maximum HR. If the maximum HR is 180 beats per minute, the target HR will be 70% of 180 = (180 × .7) = 126 beats per minute. The first two methods of calculating target HR give similar results, but the third method underestimates the target heart rate for a given MET level by approximately 15%, and must be adjusted by adding 15% to the target heart rate calculated.

For practical purposes, the target heart rate calculated by the procedures outlined previously are applicable to all the physical activities in which the individual may engage including most environmental conditions. In discontinuous exercise the alternating higher and lower energy demands may be accompanied by heart rates 10% higher or 10% lower than the prescribed target heart rate. However, the exercise intervals should be of such duration that the heart rate, over time, averages out to the prescribed level.

Heart rate can be determined from measurements made during ECG monitoring, radiotelemetry, or palpation. The latter two methods are more adaptable to non-laboratory situations, with the palpation technique better suited to large groups. Counting the pulse for 10 seconds immediately after a bout of exercise and multiplying by 6 gives a good estimation of exercise heart rate.

In a specific physical conditioning session, the exercise specialist may use the MET prescription, heart rate prescription, or both in setting appropriate exercise intensities in various activities. As one adapts to conditioning, heart rate for a given MET level will generally decrease; therefore, participants will be able to increase progressively their MET level to correspond to their target heart rate. Periodic re-evaluation will aid in measuring progress and checking the exercise prescription.

C. DURATION OF THE EXERCISE SESSION

The conditioning period will usually vary in length from 15 to 60 minutes. This length of time is required to improve functional capacity. The appropriate duration of the conditioning period is inversely related to the intensity of the exercise expressed as a percentage of functional capacity. Compared to persons with low functional capacities, persons with high functional capacities are able to maintain a higher percentage of their functional capacity for a longer period of time. The conditioning response resulting from an exercise program is a result of the interaction of the intensity and the duration of exercise. Significant cardiovascular improvements have been obtained with exercise sessions of 5 to 10 minutes' duration with an intensity of more than 90% of functional capacity. However, high intensity-short duration sessions are not desirable for most sedentary or symptomatic participants (participant categories C–H Table 1) and better results are obtained with lower intensities and longer durations.

For sedentary, asymptomatic, and symptomatic participants (participant categories C–H Table 1) exercise sessions of moderate duration (20 to 30 minutes) and moderate intensity (70 to 80% or lower of functional capacity) are advisable during the first weeks of conditioning. Changes in the exercise prescription may be made as the individual's functional capacity increases and as physiologic adaptation to exercise occurs. Modification of the duration-intensity level should be individualized on the basis of subject's functional capacity, health status, and response to specific exercise activities. If a normal conditioning response is obtained with no complications, the duration may be increased from 20 to 45 minutes after the first 2 weeks. As mentioned previously, the interaction of intensity and duration should be such that the participant experiences no undue fatigue an hour after the completion of the exercise session.

An adequate conditioning response can be elicited by maintaining a prescribed exercise intensity, or a prescribed heart rate, for a period of approximately 15 minutes per exercise session. With the inclusion of the warm-up and cool-down periods the total duration per session would be a minimum of 30 minutes. For most participants daily exercise of such duration will result in an increase in or maintenance of a desirable level of functional capacity.

D. FREQUENCY OF EXERCISE SESSIONS

The frequency of exercise will depend in part on the duration and intensity of the exercise session. The frequency will vary from several daily sessions, to 3 to 5 periods per week according to the functional capacity of the participants. The exercise program director or exercise specialist should determine the frequency of exercise for the specific requirements of participants. For some individuals with functional capacities less than 3 METS, sessions of 5 minutes several times daily may be desirable. For persons with capacities between 3 and 5 METS, 1 to 2 daily sessions may be advisable. Participants with capacities of 5 to 8 METS should exercise at least 3 times a week. Exercise sessions on alternate days are desirable if conditioning occurs less than daily.

When initiating a jogging program, excessive bone-joint stress may occur. It is desirable to alternate a day of exercise with a day of rest. Once adaptation is accomplished a greater conditioning response may be obtained by daily exercise.

E. RATE OF PROGRESSION

The progress of a participant in an exercise conditioning program depends on the progressive steps involved in the endurance or aerobic phase of the exercise program. Warm-up and cool-down phases should be adjusted in direct proportion to the duration of the endurance or aerobic phase of exercise. Progression in the exercise conditioning program is dependent on an individual's functional capacity, health status, age, and needs or goals. The endurance or aerobic phase of the exercise prescription has three stages of progression: initial, improvement, and maintenance.

1. *Initial Conditioning Stage.* The initial stage should include stretching, light calisthenics, and low level aerobic activities in which the participant will experience a minimum of muscle soreness and can avoid debilitating injuries or discomfort. Discomfort is often associated with starting an exercise program without adequate time for physiologic adaptation. It may help to start with an exercise intensity approximately 1 MET lower than that estimated at 70 to 90% of the functional capacity. By using the graded exercise test results and the calculated exercise intensity in METS, the exercise specialist or exercise program director can estimate the aerobic phase exercise intensity for different types of activity. For example, using the data in Figure 1, the exercise intensity can be set for an eventual 7 to 9 METS at a target heart rate of 144 to 168. The initial prescription might be set at a more conservative 6 METS. If the participant selects a jogging program, information in Table 4 indicates that a 5 mph pace would be appropriate. A bicycle ergometer program might also be suggested for this 70 kg participant at 600 kgm per minute (Table 5). These estimates from the Table values should always be checked in actuality by having the participant, unless symptom limited, exercise at these intensities for a minimum of 2 minutes and then checking the pulse. Exercise intensities may require adjustment; lower intensity if the participant is above the target heart rate, and greater intensity if the participant is below target heart rate. With conditioning, heart rate

decreases for a constant exercise intensity. Therefore, the heart rate (used in combination with signs and symptoms) is one of the best indicators available to indicate when to advance the participant to the next level. This may be determined by consultation among the physician, exercise program director, and exercise specialist. A combination of objective and subjective factors must be considered when progressing individuals in their exercise routines.

The total duration of the initial aerobic phase of the exercise prescription should be at least 12 minutes and gradually be increased. Frequency will depend on the initial functional capacity (p. 50) and cardiorespiratory fitness level (Table 11). The initial activities usually last from 4 to 6 weeks, but this is dependent on the adaptation of the participant to the program. For example, a person who has a fitness level ranked "fair" or is limited by CHD may spend as many as 6 to 10 weeks in the initial program, while the participant with a fitness level of "good to high" may not need to participate as long in the initial phase or may be

TABLE 11.   CARDIORESPIRATORY FITNESS LEVELS*

Fitness Level	$O_2 ml/kg \cdot min$	METS
Poor	3.5–13.9	1.0– 3.9
Low	14.0–24.9	4.0– 6.9
Average	25.0–38.9	7.0–10.9
Good	39.0–48.9	11.0–13.9
High	49.0–56.0	14.0–16.0

*For 40-year-old males. Adjustments are appropriate to apply these standards to others.

exempted from this stage if already engaged in an exercise program.

Health status must also be considered. For example, patients with symptoms of exertional angina during the initial stage may have to exercise for a period of time at 40 to 50% of functional capacity. Persons with intermittent claudication may only be able to tolerate 1 to 2 minutes of exercise alternated with rest periods. Following a debilitating illness or major surgery functional capacities are often as low as 2 to 3 METS. Initially, exercise duration may be less than 5 minutes due to angina, local muscle fatigue, or breathlessness. The necessity for individual modifications cannot be overemphasized, although no attempt can be made to provide a list of all the possible modifications for all participants.

All needs and goals of the participant should be considered when developing the progression of the aerobic phase of the exercise program. For example, those participants desiring to lose body weight should be made aware of caloric intake and energy cost of various activities in which they are engaged. A minimum energy expenditure of 300 kcal per exercise session and 1000 kcal per week is recommended for both asymptomatic and symptomatic participants. The average healthy sedentary participant (8 to 12 METS functional capacity) can usually attain the 200 kcal level per exercise session during the first week of conditioning. The average participant with steady progression can reach 300 kcal per exercise session in 8 to 12 weeks, while some cardiac patients or other symptomatic participants may require as long as 2 years. The difference between the two groups is due to the greater variability in myocardial limitations rather than in their adaptation to conditioning. Usually, increased frequency of conditioning of up to 5 to 6 days per week will greatly increase the total energy expenditure. If, as in the example, one objective of the exercise program is to obtain ideal body weight, the program design should increase caloric output. The addition of one extra 400 kcal workout per week to the conditioning regimen should remove approximately 1 pound of fat every 9 weeks. If this is matched by a similar reduction in food intake it will amount to a reduction of 12 pounds in a year. Timing the activity so as to take advantage of the brief, but often helpful, appetite inhibition immediate post-exercise may also help.

2. *Improvement Conditioning Stage.* The improvement stage of the aerobic phase of the exercise conditioning program differs from the initial stage in that the participant is progressed at a more rapid rate. During this stage the intensity level is increased to the full 70 to 90% of functional capacity and the duration is increased rather consistently every 2 to 3 weeks. How well the participant adapts to the current level of conditioning dictates the frequency and magnitude of the progression. Cardiac patients and less fit individuals should be permitted more time for adaptation at each stage of conditioning. It is recommended that symptom limited participants initially use discontinuous aerobic exercise and progress toward continuous aerobic exercise. The duration of exercise for these participants should be increased before increasing the intensity (Table 12). Age must also be taken into consideration when progressions are recommended.

TABLE 12. EXAMPLE: PROGRESSION OF THE SYMPTOMATIC PARTICIPANT USING A DISCONTINUOUS AEROBIC CONDITIONING PHASE*

Endurance/ Aerobic Phase	Weeks	Total Minutes at %FC**	%FC	Minutes at Exercise Intensity (60–80% FC)	Minutes at Rest Phase Lower than Exercise Intensity	Repetitions
Initial Stage	1	12	60	2	1	6
	2	14	60	2	1	7
	3	16	60	2	1	8
	4	18	60–70	2	1	9
	5	20	60–70	2	1	10
Improvement Stage	6–9	21	70–80	3	1	7
	10–13	24	70–80	3	1	8
	14–16	24	70–80	4	1	6
	17–19	28	70–80	4	1	7
	20–23	30	70–80	5	1	6
	24–27	30	70–80	Continuous		
Maintenance Stage	28+	45–60	70–80	Continuous		

*Clinical status must be considered before advancing to the next level
**FC—Functional Capacity

As a general rule the adaptation to conditioning takes approximately 40% longer, or an additional week, for each decade in life after age 30.

3. *Maintenance Conditioning Stage.* The maintenance stage of the exercise prescription usually begins after the first 6 months of training. During the maintenance stage the participant usually reaches a satisfactory level of cardiorespiratory fitness and may be no longer interested in increasing the conditioning load. While further improvement may be minimal, continuing the same workout schedule enables one to maintain fitness.

At this point the objectives of conditioning should be reviewed and realistic goals set. To maintain fitness a specific exercise program should be designed that will be similar in caloric cost to the initial program and also satisfy the needs of the participant over a long time span. More enjoyable or variable activities may be substituted for the improvement stage activities of walking and jogging. This may help avoid participant dropouts which result from activities which become boring due to repetition. The important point is that participation in activities that are enjoyed is more likely to be continued.

4

Types of Exercise Programs

Medical evaluation and graded exercise testing permit the classification of participants according to their capacity for participation in an unsupervised or supervised exercise program.

A. UNSUPERVISED EXERCISE PROGRAMS

Asymptomatic participants with functional capacities of 8 METS or more can usually exercise safely in an unsupervised conditioning program (participant categories A–C Table 1). Participant safety can be enhanced by individualizing the exercise prescription, having knowledge of the energy cost of various activities, and an awareness of the physiologic effects of temperature, humidity, and altitude on exercising.

B. SUPERVISED EXERCISE PROGRAMS

Supervised exercise programs are initially advisable for asymptomatic participants with functional capacities less than 8 METS, participants with known CHD risk factors (participant category D), and for cardiorespiratory patients regardless of their functional capacities (participant categories E, F, G, H).

Prior to participation in a supervised exercise program all participants must sign an informed consent document (Appendix E).

Activities undertaken in supervised exercise programs will vary depending upon the functional capacity and health status of the participants. These programs should be under the combined guidance of a physician and an exercise program director or exercise specialist. Direct supervision of each session by a physician is not required in a supervised activity program, but the attendance of qualified personnel is mandatory.

Although types of supervised exercise programs vary because of locale, available facilities, and staff, four distinct programs can be identified: in-patient; out-patient; home, and community based programs.

1. *In-Patient Exercise Programs.* The in-patient exercise program is frequently offered for post-myocardial, postoperative cardiovascular, pulmonary disease patients and other patient groups that may benefit from such services while in the hospital. The in-patient program usually includes supervised ambulatory therapy. Contraindications for patients participating in ambulatory exercise are consistent with contraindications for performing a graded exercise test (see Chapter 2). However, termination points for exercise should be more conservative than those outlined for terminating the graded exercise test. These generally include that the heart rate should not exceed certain limits, that ST-segment displacement on the ECG indicative of myocardial ischemia and/or arrhythmias are minimal during ambulation. The exercise should not induce angina, palpitations, dyspnea,

or excessive fatigue. ECG monitoring equipment for determining appropriate exercise responses must be available. The staff-patient ratio is generally 1:1. An emergency team is available in the area. The in-patient program may include a predischarge submaximal or symptom-limited graded exercise test which may aid the physician in providing better patient management and follow-up. The goals of the in-patient exercise program are to return patients to daily physical activities and to begin patient education involving required life-style changes which set the stage for later cardiac rehabilitation.

2. *Out-Patient Exercise Programs.* The out-patient exercise program provides a continuation of the in-patient program and usually begins immediately after hospital discharge. These participants usually have a functional capacity of at least 3 METS. This exercise program should be prescribed, regularly scheduled, and supervised. ECG monitoring capabilities must be available and may be used on a scheduled basis or as needed. The patients' functional capacity, symptoms, or ECG limitations determine the staff-patient ratio, which may vary from a 1:1 to a 1:10 ratio. The program is the responsibility of a physician who may be in attendance regularly or on call. The goals of the out-patient program are to provide physical rehabilitation for resumption of habitual and occupational activities and to continue patient education for life-style changes.

3. *Home Exercise Programs.* Characteristics of a home exercise program are similar to an out-patient program. However, symptomatic and asymptomatic participants may be included. In addition to exercising

at home the participant may return to the out-patient program for scheduled, monitored reevaluation of the exercise prescription. The type of exercise prescribed is based on patients' functional capacity, symptoms, and ECG changes. In addition, exercise equipment available and personal preference should be considered. Ideally, those with functional capacities of 3 to 5 METS should be placed on a controlled exercise program. Walking according to a time-distance heart-rate protocol or pedaling a bicycle ergometer at a given load and pulse-rate is recommended. Home programs designed for persons with functional capacities of more than 5 METS may include more diverse activities. When possible, symptomatic participants should be required to participate in the out-patient program prior to exercising at home.

4. *Community Exercise Programs.* Participants in community exercise programs may have progressed through hospital, in-patient, and out-patient programs or may have been referred without previous participation. These programs may accept patients with a variety of cardiorespiratory problems, depending on clinical judgment, facilities, equipment, and availability of qualified staff. The community based exercise program may include patients who are approximately 6 to 8 weeks post-infarction, 4 to 8 weeks post-cardiac surgery, have clinically stable or decreasing angina, and have arrhythmias under reasonable control during exercise. Frequently, pulmonary patients and those with incomplete responsive hypertension may also benefit from such programs. Admission criteria vary and must be based on clinical and policy judgments. The community program provides an on-going mainte-

nance program in which patients generally stay a minimum of 6 months. The suggested minimum functional capacity of participants in the community program is 5 METS but patients with a lower MET capacity may be admitted depending on local circumstances. Community programs are not generally located in clinical settings but may be offered three or more times per week in community facilities. An effective community program requires a minimum of two certified staff members, standing orders for emergency procedures, emergency equipment, and an on-call emergency team, and a staff-patient ratio of 1:10. It is advisable to train participants in CPR. Electrocardiographic monitoring can be performed in a community setting but this requires additional staff and equipment.

Efforts should be made to move participants gradually to programs with less supervision. Participants who prove that they can self-regulate their exercise programs should be given increased freedom to do so. The graded exercise test and medical evaluation should be continued on a 3 to 6 month basis and eventually limited to a yearly occurrence or as needed.

C. PARTICIPANT EXIT

Exit criteria for participants from the community program include the following:

1. The participant should have attained a functional capacity of 8 METS or greater.
2. The ECG taken at rest prior to exit should be the same as or improved when compared with the

resting ECG taken at entry to the exercise conditioning program.

3. The ECG taken at maximum exercise should be within normal limits or show stabilization of PR or QRS conduction patterns and ST changes.

4. Symptoms of angina or dyspnea should be stable or absent at maximum exercise levels or at exercise levels adequate to maintain the patient's necessary life-style.

5. Resting blood pressure and heart rate should be within normal limits not exceeding a blood pressure reading of 160/96 and a resting heart rate of 90 beats per minute.

6. Participants should understand the basic pathophysiology of their disease, effects of their present medication, and the need for continued life-style changes.

Evaluation of participants' status by the physician, the exercise program director, and the exercise specialist should determine the readiness for exit from a program. Clinical signs such as persistent post-exercise dyspnea, undue fatigue or depression, exercise anxiety, unchanged angina levels, exercise induced CNS symptoms, rapid weight gain, or musculoskeletal problems may indicate that the participant is not ready for exit from the program. Participants with these conditions should be referred to the physician for further evaluation. Participants who do not demonstrate normal progress may be identified by a subsequent graded exercise test. Measurements made during a subsequent graded exercise test that substantiate a lack of normal progress in response to a conditioning program are: (1) no change or an increase in heart rate and blood pressure and pulse-pressure product responses to the same submaximal exercise intensities; (2) a decrease in systolic blood pressures with increasing exercise intensities; (3) significant symptoms or ECG changes occurring at the same or lower submaximal levels than before exercise conditioning, and (4) a decrease in $\dot{V}O_2$ max or functional capacity.

D. SPECIAL CONSIDERATIONS FOR EXERCISE PROGRAMS

The process of exercise prescription involves developing a balanced program which has the potential for improving the functional capacity of a specific individual. When the individual has identified medical problems or diagnosed disease, the exercise prescription must be modified to enable the participant with special circumstances to make the best physiologic and psychologic adjustment to the conditioning program.

1. *Exercise Prescription for the Patient With Angina Pectoris.* Patients with stable angina are excellent candidates for exercise programs. The object of physical conditioning in the patient with angina is to increase the amount of exercise performed before the onset of limiting angina. The patient must be evaluated for ischemic responses before, during, and after the graded exercise test. An essential element of this evaluation is the patient's description of the anginal episodes. This evaluation should include: *(a)* verbal description of symptoms (e.g., discomfort, pressure,

tightness, burning, shortness of breath); *(b)* location of symptoms (e.g., substernal, jaw, teeth, throat, interscapular area, elbow, arm, wrist, epigastrium); *(c)* observed actions of the patient (e.g., clenched fist, rubbing); *(d)* duration and frequency of the episodes; *(e)* precipitating factors (e.g., rest, exertion, emotion); and *(f)* methods used to relieve the angina (e.g., rest, nitroglycerin). Palpation of the painful chest area may help in differentiating musculoskeletal chest pain from that of the true angina. Teaching the patient to grade the angina symptom during the exercise test may be beneficial in determining the intensity of the discomfort for test termination (+3) and to judge exertion end points (+2) (see p. 24).

Many patients with angina experience the onset of symptoms at low levels of exercise, i.e., 2 or 3 METS. Graded exercise test protocols beginning at 1.5 or 2 METS help to identify onset of angina for these patients. Medication or exercise conditioning may produce subtle changes in MET capacity, heart rate, and blood pressure responses of patients with angina. Graded exercise test protocols of 0.5 MET increments may reflect these changes. Initial testing without drugs is helpful in estimating the magnitude of the ischemic response. Patients on antianginal medications whose functional capacity is being evaluated for exercise prescription should continue medications as usual. Administration of nitrates during the exercise test may add information for the exercise prescription. If propranolol is prescribed following evaluation of the diagnostic test, the graded exercise test should be repeated when the maintenance dosage is achieved. This re-evaluation will establish the patient's medicated response during exercise and allow a more accurate exercise prescription.

Conditioning at an exercise level equivalent to 70 to 85% of that provoking angina at a frequency and duration described in Chapter 3 should elicit the desired conditioning responses. The exact exercise intensity may be determined by the type of program in which the patient is participating, supervised or unsupervised. The expected ischemic, arrhythmic, and anginal responses at specific conditioning intensities should be noted in the exercise prescription.

For the patient with angina who is not on medication, the exercise session should begin with a prolonged warm-up of at least 10 minutes' duration. After the warm-up, the aerobic phase of the exercise session can begin. Patients with angina may benefit from intermittent exercise in which exercising at prescribed intensities is followed by rest periods. This arrangement may be continued until the patient with angina has sufficient strength and stamina to sustain continuous exercise. An effort should be made to utilize all major muscle groups, including the upper extremities. It is especially important to emphasize dynamic repetitive motions and to eliminate any tendency toward breath-holding. Patients should be cautioned not to exercise through angina when the discomfort continues to increase beyond a +2 intensity level. Rather, the patient should decrease activity until the discomfort subsides before continuing exercise at the previous intensity. Cool-down should be gradual and prolonged, at least 10 minutes, to prevent complications created by hydrostatic blood pooling in the lower extremities. Caution should be used when supervising patients for whom prophylactic use of nitroglycerin or long acting nitrates has been prescribed before or during exercise. Adverse hypotensive responses may occur in these patients, especially if they are taking other medications which may cause a decrease in blood pressure, (e.g., antiarrhythmics, beta-blockers—propranolol, diuretics—hydrochlorothiazide). If exertional angina is not relieved by terminating exercise or by the use of 3 sublingual nitroglycerin tablets (1 taken every 5 minutes), the patient should be stabilized and prepared for transport to the nearest adequate hospital emergency room.

2. *Exercise Prescription for the Cardiac Patient With Diabetes Mellitus.* Diabetes mellitus is frequently found in patients who have had myocardial infarctions or circulatory problems of the lower extremities due to the accelerated atherosclerosis associated with diabetes. Two potential problems occur in exercising insulin-medicated diabetics. The first problem is that lack of sufficient insulin may cause a hyperglycemic effect in the blood because cellular absorption of glucose is restricted. A second problem is the hypoglycemic effect which occurs due to an increased mobilization of depot insulin, particularly if the injection site was in the exercising muscle. Since physical activity has an insulin-like effect, the exercise program requires an insulin-dependent diabetic to either reduce insulin intake or increase carbohydrate intake. It is important to instruct the diabetic participant and the exercise staff that during prolonged activities adequate nourishment must be available in the form of sugar, fruit juice, and/or other readily digestible carbohydrates. The exercise program director and the exercise

specialist should be aware of any participants who are diabetic and their hypoglycemic symptoms. Special attention should be paid to patients taking insulin and beta-blocker medication as the hypoglycemic symptoms may be masked.

3. *Exercise Prescription for the Cardiac Patient Who Has Claudication Pain.* Individuals with significant peripheral vascular disease are at a much higher risk of having associated coronary and cerebral vascular disease than those without peripheral impairment. Intermittent testing protocols may be advantageous when evaluating these patients for exercise. Subjective gradation of pain is a useful technique for expressing claudication discomfort and can be divided into the following general categories:

Grade IV—Excruciating and unbearable pain.
Grade III—Intense pain (short of Grade IV) from which the patient's attention cannot be diverted except by catastrophic events (i.e., fire, explosion).
Grade II— Moderate discomfort or pain from which the patient's attention can be diverted by a number of common stimuli (i.e., conversation, an interesting episode on T.V.).
Grade I— Definite discomfort or pain but only of initial or modest level (established—but minimal).

Activity should consist of an aerobic activity at least daily (a minimum of 5 days a week), and preferably with two periods of exercise per day. Activities might include walking, stationary bicycling, swimming or pool activities where the patient is exercised in shallow warm water. Intensity of exercise must be balanced between the Grade II pain level and the prescribed target heart rate. The duration of each exercise session should be at least 20 minutes.

4. *Exercise Prescription for the Cardiac Patient Who Has Concomitant Pulmonary Disease.* Although it has been demonstrated that aerobic exercise fails to improve indices of pulmonary function, exercise may improve cardiovascular function, and does improve skeletal muscle strength and endurance. These improvements will reduce the demands on limited pulmonary reserve during effort.

Patients suspected of having pulmonary disease should be assessed by a respiratory physician clinically and with appropriate pulmonary function tests. It is helpful to screen all cardiac patients entering an exercise program with simple spirometry measurements, vital capacity (VC), and volume expired in the first second of a forced expiration (FEV_1). Any patient found to have VC or FEV_1 which is less than 80% of predicted values should be referred to his physician for advice before undergoing exercise testing, so that appropriate measurements may be made.

Graded exercise test protocols may be continuous or discontinuous. With the limited work capacity often associated with pulmonary disease, small increases in work load are recommended. The patient is likely to achieve a higher maximal exercise rate in a graded exercise test in which the time spent at each work rate is short. The most common reason patients give for discontinuing the test is dyspnea. Essential variables to be measured during the graded exercise test, in addition to ECG and blood pressure, include ventilation, respiratory frequency, and tidal volume. Other important information may be obtained from oxygen consumption, carbon dioxide output, and non-invasive measurement of the arterial oxygen saturation (SaO_2). Arterial blood gas analysis may be important in patients with gas exchange disturbances.

Ideally the exercise prescription should be determined in consultation with the referring physician, and should take into account the degree of respiratory disability as assessed clinically, through pulmonary function tests, and on the graded exercise test. Patients with mild degrees of pulmonary dysfunction may not be limited by a reduced ventilatory capacity and may be dealt with in the same way as other cardiac patients. Patients who are significantly limited by pulmonary factors should not be enrolled in the program until therapy is judged to be optimal by the physician. Some patients will require medication before or during activity. This applies particularly to patients with exercise induced bronchoconstriction. Prescribed endurance activity should not lead to a ventilatory response greater than about 80% of the maximum ventilation attained in the graded exercise test. Patients who exhibit an abnormal breathing pattern during the graded exercise test may be helped by advice regarding proper breathing techniques. Some severely limited patients may require supplemental oxygen during activity if this has been objectively demonstrated by graded exercise testing to improve exercise performance. It is recommended that supplemental oxygen should be administered through a high flow O_2 enrichment system giving an inspired O_2

concentration of 24 or 28%. The advice of a respiratory therapist may be valuable in this regard.

Modifications in the duration of exercise may be required; for example, two 10-minute sessions or even four 5-minute sessions daily. As an individual's tolerance for exercise improves, the duration or intensity of each session may progressively increase. The type of exercise is essentially the same as for cardiac patients. Brisk walking, jogging, and cycling are useful activities. Swimming techniques, modified by the use of swim fins and a kickboard, also may be useful. Upper body aerobic exercise, such as rowing and arm cranking are generally not applicable because of the high ventilation required at a given power output in this type of exercise.

5. *Exercise Prescription for the Cardiac Patient Who Has Arthritis.* Exercise producing excess stress on osteoarthritic joints should be avoided. A specific exercise program should be performed daily to maintain and improve both range of joint motion and muscle strength. Exercises should not be severely painful, but slight pain may be tolerated. Exercise periods of short duration and increasing frequency impose less stress on osteoarthritic joints.

Cardiac patients who have rheumatoid arthritis are limited in their ability to adhere to a specific exercise regimen because of the complication arising from the arthritic problem. Weight bearing activities, for example, are contraindicated during inflammatory episodes in the lower extremities. However, every effort must be made to sustain satisfactory levels of muscular strength and range of joint motion.

For many patients with osteo- or rheumatoid arthritis a walk-jog program might be stressful. Alternatives to the walk-jog exercise program include cycling, arm-ergometry, and rowing. Swimming is often recommended as an acceptable exercise. The intensity of a swimming exercise prescription depends upon the patients' proficiency in the water, their ability to modify swimming strokes to minimize the stress to the affected joints, and their target heart rates.

6. *Exercise Prescription for the Obese Cardiac Patient.* Many patients with cardiac problems are 20% above optimal body weight as determined by indirect methods of body fat assessment. These obese patients present special problems in graded exercise testing. If locomotion on the motor driven treadmill is not possible, a bicycle ergometer should be used to test functional capacity.

An exercise prescription for the obese patient should be of low intensity and prolonged duration. Orthopedic problems particularly of the hip, knee, and ankle can be avoided if the intensity of exercise is low and sustained over time (40 to 60 minutes). Exercise apparel that includes proper footwear is essential. Obese patients are more prone to conditions that may lead to syncope during an exercise session. This response occurs due to fluid imbalance resulting from dietary restrictions and exercise induced fluid loss. Syncope can be alleviated by having the obese subject assume the hook lying supine position during the cool-down phase of the exercise session.

7. *Exercise Prescription for the Cardiac Patient Who Has Low Back Pain.* Special routines should be performed by the cardiac patient with low back problems. Exercises of a prophylactic nature which

strengthen the abdominals and relax the back extensor muscles should be performed daily. Isometric contractions with breath holding or exercises inducing pain are to be avoided.

8. *Exercise Prescription for Stress Management in Cardiac Rehabilitation.* Stress management techniques (e.g., progressive relaxation, quieting responses) can be initiated during the recuperation period following myocardial infarction and integrated into the exercise conditioning program. Relaxation techniques conducted immediately after the cool-down phase of each exercise session may prove beneficial. If used independently of the exercise sessions, 10 to 20 minutes several times a day is often sufficient to achieve the desired results.

9. *Exercise Prescription for the Elderly Cardiac Patient.* Since the majority of the elderly suffer from one or more chronic diseases, appropriate modifications should be applied to the exercise prescription. A decrease in range of motion, flexibility, muscular strength, functional capacity, and an increased bone degeneration occurs with aging and a sedentary lifestyle. These physiologic changes may be offset with exercise intensities as low as 40% with a duration of 20 to 30 minutes and a frequency of 3 times per week.

5

Exercise Program Administration

The growth of exercise programs and the diversity among them have created a need for administrative guidelines. The following general administrative guidelines are applicable to exercise programs.

A. MANAGEMENT—STRUCTURE AND FUNCTION

Effective program administration is enhanced through well-defined organizational relationships which clearly identify specific personnel responsibilities and sources of authority. Ultimate accountability for the program should rest with a governing body/advisory committee composed of appropriate professionals who contribute their collective knowledge toward development and operation of the program. The policies and procedures adopted by this body provide the guidelines for developing and operating the exercise program and the delegation of responsibilities to appropriate administrators. Good administration fosters constructive communication and provides a way of evaluating program effectiveness and initiating appropriate changes.

The position of an exercise program administrator requires training and experience in leadership, planning, delegation of authority, and assumption of responsibility. The effective administrator has a broad academic understanding, insight into human relationships, practical intelligence, and a strong commitment to exercise program goals.

B.   FINANCIAL CONCERNS

Income and expenditure accounting procedures are established within guidelines determined by the program governing board. A board member with accounting capabilities will facilitate development of practical policies. Some financial planning is assured by a realistic and accurate appraisal of conditions affecting the program. Budget development should follow a reasonable sequence which includes inventory, staff input, analysis and review, submission and approval, revision and budget administration. Regular income sources must be managed carefully to ensure a consistent cash flow in balance with projected expenses.

The major source of income for preventive and rehabilitative exercise programs is through participants' fees. These exercise programs should use materials which explain the program fees to the participant and the insurance carriers prior to enrollment. Medicare, Medicaid, and Vocational Rehabilitation agencies should be considered as alternate income sources. Additional sources of income in the form of grants should be identified, developed, and utilized. Such income may be reserved for research, financial contingencies, and capital expenditures. Line item accountability is the most accurate method of bookkeeping and with standard record keeping practices provides reliable data for future financial planning.

C. LEGAL CONSIDERATIONS

It is essential that approved program procedures or standing orders be developed through careful study of national and local practices and with the guidance of medical and legal advisors to provide the best standards of reasonable and prudent care. Constant scrutiny of supervisory personnel, activity selection, and/or environmental conditions along with regular in-service training of staff should be provided within these standards. Specific policies for protection of the rights and safety of patients must be developed and understood by all staff persons. Such policies include, but are not limited to, the obtaining of informed consent, the basis of which provides documentation of the voluntary assumption of risk by the participant.

Administrators must be aware that state statutes which govern the practice of medicine are generally restrictive, vary widely in scope and, if violated, can result in criminal prosecution. Self-protective procedures include in-service training to keep abreast of current accepted procedures, employing certified or licensed staff persons, periodic recertification of personnel, securing satisfactory limits of liability insurance, careful screening of participants, and procedures for elimination of participants who cannot safely be managed in an exercise program.

D. FACILITY AND EQUIPMENT REQUIREMENTS

Careful matching of program activities, facilities, and equipment will contribute to the continued success of an exercise program. The ideal facility requirements for a program include: *(a)* a walking-running area with safe traffic patterns; *(b)* a testing area which is quiet, electrically grounded, and offers easy access for emergency situations; *(c)* an educational area in which lectures, demonstrations, films, and study materials can be made available; *(d)* a private counseling area; *(e)* an administrative area in which records and other office materials are secure; and *(f)* locker rooms and restrooms which are well ventilated, easily accessible, secure, and supervised.

Specific equipment and supply requirements are determined by the type of program offered. The administrator should maintain records of suppliers, warranty agreements, operating manuals, replacement availabilities, and costs. A complete preventive maintenance program that includes calibration checks is recommended for optimal equipment performance. Local fire codes and regulations should be posted along with emergency evacuation routes. All staff personnel should be held responsible for educating participants and enforcing the safe use of facilities and equipment in accordance with procedures approved by the governing body.

Suggested reading material:

1. Specifications for Exercise Testing Equipment. *Circulation (59)* 849A-854A; April, 1979.

E. PUBLIC RELATIONS

The function of public relations is to influence opinion through communications with the community and participants. Public relations includes publicity, advertising, and promotion. It is essentially an administrative responsibility to evaluate attitudes and to identify interest in, and promote community understanding of the exercise program. Information disseminated must be timely, accurate, and comprehensible if it is to positively reflect the program. Carefully planned public relations will enable the administrator to identify community resources and obstacles. These data are essential for coordinating program efforts and interagency cooperation. Community service organizations can provide the speaking engagements and informal contacts for distributing program information which may lead to potential sources of funding. News letters, radio, television, workshops, seminars, news releases, and demonstration projects are excellent media for presenting ideas, securing new participants, and describing current events. Probably the most influential source of public relations is through participants' word-of-mouth. Though this source is not directly controllable, it is best developed through high quality program administration and through the professionalism displayed during program operations.

F. PROGRAM EVALUATION

Program evaluation is an ongoing administrative function that should be developed from several sources. Initially, the administrator should evaluate program effectiveness in terms of cost, staff productivity, public image and, most importantly, service to the participants and community. This evaluation is usually influenced by objective and subjective input from the program staff with final evaluation the responsibility of the program governing body. Second, the participants should be required to provide an evaluation of program effectiveness. Attitude assessments are useful supplements to the usual physiologic measurements included in most programs. The third source of evaluation is the input from non-participating community persons.

Effective administration is an essential component of a successful preventive or rehabilitative exercise program.

6

The Role of Physicians in Exercise Programs

Physicians have important roles in preventive and rehabilitative exercise programs. In such programs, their roles may be as leaders, support personnel, or both. In either role, physicians involved in exercise programs must be licensed to practice in the jurisdiction involved and should be protected by appropriate professional liability insurance. They should periodically be recertified in advanced cardiac life support techniques or an equivalent. Physicians must know and be able to initiate emergency and evacuation procedures appropriate to patient care.

Required competencies include the screening of persons prior to exercise and the administration of graded exercise testing. Physicians must be able to recognize electrocardiographic signs such as arrhythmias, myocardial ischemia, and evolving patterns of infarction and make decisions for patient management. Physicians must be proficient in the administration and the evaluation of responses to and side effects of various drugs commonly used by cardiorespiratory patients. They will need to understand pharmacologic mechanisms and the influence of exercise upon these actions, particularly those that influence emergency procedures. Physicians must be aware of the hazards associated with physical activities including the early signs and symptoms of dysfunction before, during, and after exercise. They must be able to record and communicate to the primary or referring physicians the data indicating dysfunction and to suggest the nature of further evaluations.

In leadership positions, physicians are diagnosticians, decision makers, teachers, counselors, and public relations persons. The physician is responsible for policies regarding the safety and clinical well-being of participants. Although this is their primary responsibility, the physician may participate with the rehabilitative team to develop and implement the exercise program. In the development of a team-approach, physicians must recognize the professional skills and competencies of exercise program directors, exercise specialists, and exercise test technologists and delegate appropriate responsibilities. Physicians should direct and participate in emergency management programs and provide continuing education for the program staff. Success of the exercise program depends upon effective communications for which the physicians' involvement and cooperation are central.

Physicians may also perform important functions in supportive roles, including their presence at graded exercise tests and exercise conditioning sessions. The guidelines recommend the circumstances during which physicians should supervise graded exercise tests. Physician attendance at specific exercise sessions is a question to be settled locally.

Ideally, a preventive and rehabilitative exercise program is initiated in a community through the leadership of physicians, an exercise program director, exercise specialists, and other allied health personnel. If local physicians have only the skills and interests required for a supporting role, a program may be initiated by an exercise program director or exercise specialist. Under these circumstances, physician guidance of the exercise program may be obtained through the development of a Medical Advisory Committee, a component of the governing body recommended for program administration.

Many physicians have been certified as Exercise Program Directors and as Exercise Specialists, but certification is not considered a necessary prerequisite for those who wish to assume medical direction of programs. The American College of Sports Medicine does not evaluate the professional expertise or competence of physicians. This role is appropriately that of the American Board of Medical Specialties and similar certifying organizations in other countries.

7

Certification of Preventive and Rehabilitative Exercise Program Personnel

There are certain functions which include specific knowledges, skills, and competencies for each of the three categories of certification: (1) exercise test technologist, (2) exercise specialist, and (3) exercise program director. There are progressive levels of knowledges, skills, and competencies required within each of the categories of certification. The exercise test technologist must demonstrate competence in graded exercise testing; the exercise specialist, in addition to the competency expected of the exercise test technologist, must demonstrate competence in executing an exercise prescription and in leading exercise; the exercise program director, in addition to the competencies expected of the exercise test technologist and exercise specialist, must demonstrate competence in administering preventive and rehabilitative programs, designing and implementing exercise programs, educating the staff and community, and designing and conducting research.

Minimal competencies have been outlined according to behavioral objectives. A behavioral objective is a statement indicating what a person should be able to do following some unit of instruction or study. Two types of objectives are presented here. The General Objective (GO) describes the unobservable mental process while the Specific Learning Objective (SLO) describes the behavior in observable terms (Table 13).

A. PREVENTIVE AND REHABILITATIVE EXERCISE TEST TECHNOLOGIST

The primary responsibility of the exercise test technologist is to administer graded exercise tests safely in order to obtain reliable and valid data. The exercise test technologist should demonstrate appropriate knowledge of functional anatomy, exercise physiology, pathophysiology, electrocardiography, and psychology in order to perform tasks such as preparing the graded exercise test station for administration of graded exercise tests, preliminary screening of the participant for the graded exercise test, administering tests and recording data, implementing emergency procedures when necessary, summarizing test data, and communicating the test results to exercise specialists, program directors, and physicians.

After participant's medical evaluation is received from a referring physician the exercise test technologist may administer a graded exercise test independently or under the supervision of a physician. This decision is based on the health status and age of the participant (Chap. 1). The technologist must be able to recognize contraindications to graded exercise testing found in preliminary screening and recognize abnormal responses during the graded exercise test and during recovery.

TABLE 13. SUMMARY OF THE FUNCTIONS, KNOWLEDGES, AND INTERNSHIP REQUIREMENTS FOR EACH PROGRESSIVE LEVEL OF CERTIFICATION

	Exercise Test Technologist	*Exercise Specialist*	*Exercise Program Director*
A. *Knowledges*			
Functional Anatomy	X	X	X
Exercise Physiology	X	X	X
Pathophysiology	X	X	X
Electrocardiography	X	X	X
Human Behavior/Psychology	X	X	X
Gerontology	X	X	X
B. *Functions*			
Exercise Testing	X	X	X
Emergency Procedures	X	X	X
Exercise Prescription		X	X
Exercise Leadership		X	X
Program Administration			X
C. *Intership**		6 Months (Approximately 800 hrs)	1 Year (Approximately 1600 hrs)

*ACSM reserves the right to modify internship requirements.

While there are no prerequisite experiences or level of education requirements for the exercise test technologist, study in the fields of the biological sciences, physical education, and health related professions are examples of appropriate training for those desiring certification. Although not mandatory, work experience under a physician or exercise program director would be a valuable asset to the certification applicant. The certified exercise test technologist working with individual participants during graded exercise and assisting in other roles in preventive and rehabilitative exercise programs may gain the necessary experience to apply for the exercise specialist certification.

Exercise Test Technologists

Behavioral Objectives. The exercise test technologist will demonstrate competency in graded exercise testing. This includes the following general and specific learning outcomes:

1. *Graded Exercise Test Administration*
   GO The exercise test technologist will demonstrate and have knowledge in administering a graded exercise test including but not limited to equipment calibration, patient screening, selecting test protocol, recording test data, data reduction, and case summary.
   SLO Describe the technique used to calibrate a motor driven treadmill, bicycle ergometer, electrocardiographic recorder, and mercury or anaeroid sphygmomanometer.

SLO Perform a routine screening procedure prior to testing. Procedures include history taking (particularly facts relevant to graded exercise test); obtaining informed consent; explaining procedures and protocol for the graded exercise test; recognizing the contraindications to a graded exercise test; providing results of screening procedures to the physician.

SLO Perform routine tasks prior to exercise testing, including:

    A. Taking a standard 12 lead electrocardiogram on a participant in a supine posture, in an upright posture, and during hyperventilation;

    B. Accurately recording right and left arm arterial blood pressure in different body postures.

SLO Perform an exercise test.

    A. Structure a graded exercise test protocol (continuous or discontinuous) with reference to the initial (starting) exercise intensity in METS, and increments of exercise intensity in METS for both the bicycle ergometer and treadmill according to the participant's age, sex, weight, estimated level of fitness, and health status.

    B. Record appropriate measurements and participant responses, e.g., symptoms, blood pressure, heart rate, and ECG at appropriate intervals during the test.

    C. Identify possible test end points or inappropriate responses which would terminate the graded exercise test.

      D. Describe post-testing procedures including cool down, stabilization of the participant, and instructions to the participant concerning showering.

      E. Demonstrate procedures used between testing sessions including turning off or putting recorders on standby and cleaning and sterilizing equipment according to routine procedures.

SLO Calculate and organize test data in a sequential manner.

      A. Transform or reduce data for the physician, program director, or exercise specialist.

GO The exercise test technologist will demonstrate knowledge in exercise testing administration.

SLO Describe a plan for organizing an exercise testing laboratory and include facilities and equipment.

SLO Describe a plan outlining the events of a typical testing day's activities.

2. *Emergency Procedures*

GO The exercise test technologist will demonstrate competency in responding, with the appropriate emergency procedures, to situations which might arise prior, during, and after the administration of graded exercise tests.

SLO Present valid CPR certification credentials.

SLO List emergency equipment which should be present in an exercise testing laboratory.

SLO Identify emergency drugs which should be available during exercise testing and demonstrate ability to assist a physician during an emergency situation.

SLO Demonstrate competency in operating and maintaining emergency equipment.

SLO Design and update emergency procedures for a preventive and rehabilitative exercise testing program.

3. *Functional Anatomy*

GO The exercise test technologist will demonstrate a knowledge of functional anatomy.

SLO Identify anatomic sites for selected measures associated with the graded exercise test.

    A. Locate the appropriate sites for the limb and chest leads of the ECG.

    B. Locate the brachial artery and position the cuff for the measurement of blood pressure.

    C. Locate anatomic landmarks that might be required in determining the peripheral pulses.

    D. Locate anatomic landmarks that might be required in anthropometry.

    E. Locate the anatomic landmarks used during cardiopulmonary resuscitation and emergency procedures.

4. *Exercise Physiology*

GO The exercise test technologist will demonstrate a knowledge of exercise physiology.

SLO Define aerobic and anaerobic metabolism.

SLO List the normal cardiorespiratory responses

to the graded exercise test including heart rate (HR), stroke volume (SV), cardiac output ($\dot{Q}$), blood pressure (BP), ventilation ($\dot{V}_E$).

SLO List modifications to graded exercise testing.

    A. List physiologic considerations in the selection of different modes of ergometry, i.e., treadmill, bicycle, or arm ergometer.

    B. Describe the principle of specificity as it relates to the mode of testing.

    C. List the advantages and disadvantages of continuous vs. discontinuous tests.

    D. Describe the physiologic importance of the warm-up, rate of progression, and cool-down aspects of graded exercise testing.

    E. List the effects of temperature and humidity upon the physiologic response to graded exercise testing.

    F. List the signs and symptoms that are used in designating the endpoint of a graded exercise test.

5. *Pathophysiology*

    GO The exercise test technologist will demonstrate a knowledge of the basic pathophysiology of CHD.

    SLO Define ischemia and explain the methods that are used to record and measure ischemic responses. List the effects of a myocardial infarction upon performance and safety during a graded exercise test.

    SLO Define hypotension and hypertension.

    SLO List major risk factors for CHD.

SLO Explain why blood pressure should be monitored during the graded exercise test.

SLO List special considerations necessary when testing participants with obesity, diabetes, asthma, orthopedic, or neurologic problems.

SLO List the major drugs which might affect the graded exercise test results.

6. *Electrocardiography*

GO The exercise test technologist will demonstrate a knowledge of normal and abnormal resting electrocardiograms and be able to recognize selected ECG abnormalities during the administration of a graded exercise test.

SLO Describe the normal resting electrocardiogram.

    A. Draw a normal ECG complex and label important waves, intervals, and points.

    B. List functional phenomena or events associated with the various segments of the electrocardiogram.

SLO Identify the ECG changes that are associated with an ischemic response at rest and during exercise.

    A. Draw and label an ECG complexs that is representative of an ischemic response, subendocardial and transmural.

    B. Define the limits or considerations in terminating a graded exercise test (or continuing the recovery) on the basis of an ischemic response.

SLO Identify the ECG changes that are associated with the following abnormalities: arrhythmias; conduction defects; myocardial infarctions.

A. Draw and label ECG complexes that are representative of the following abnormalities:
1. Myocardial infarction.
2. Cardiac standstill (ventricular asystole).
3. Bradycardia ($\leq$60/min).
4. Differences between supraventricular and ventricular rhythms.
5. Premature ventricular complexes (frequency, multifocal, and R on T).
6. Ventricular tachycardia.
7. Ventricular fibrillation.
8. Atrioventricular blocks of all degrees.
9. Atrial fibrillation.
10. Atrial flutter.

B. Define the limits or considerations in terminating a graded exercise test (or continuing the recovery) on the basis of the ECG abnormalities listed.

7. *Human Behavior/Psychology*

GO The exercise test technologist will demonstrate knowledge of psychologic factors affecting exercise testing environments.

SLO List six factors which increase anxiety in the exercise testing laboratory.

SLO Describe how anxiety may be reduced in a participant.

8. *Gerontology*

GO The exercise test technologist will demonstrate competence in selecting appropriate test protocol for the older participant.

SLO Describe adjustments which might be necessary for testing the older participant, specifically, instructions for the patient and modification of the testing protocol and testing equipment.

B. PREVENTIVE AND REHABILITATIVE EXERCISE SPECIALIST

Exercise appears to have an appropriate and accepted role in preventive and rehabilitative medical programs. The unique competency of the preventive and rehabilitative exercise specialist is the ability to lead exercise for persons with medical limitations, especially cardiorespiratory and related diseases, as well as leading exercise for healthy asymptomatic populations. The exercise specialist, in conjunction with the exercise program director or physician, must be able to design an exercise prescription based on graded exercise test results, evaluate participants' responses to exercise and conditioning, assist in the education of patients, and interact and communicate effectively with the physician, exercise program director, exercise test technologist, program participants, and with the community at large.

The exercise specialist must demonstrate the competencies required of the exercise test technologist. Curricula that enhance the preparation for the position of exercise specialist include, but are not limited to, exercise physiology and the health related and allied health professions. An internship of at least 6 months (approximately 800 hours) is required before applying for certification. This internship should be under the direction of a physician or exercise program director and include a variety of experiences including graded exercise testing, prescription, and supervision of individual and group exercise programs for *participants with medically diagnosed disease or limitations, particularly cardiac disease.*

An exercise specialist in activity programs for prevention and rehabilitation of individuals with medical or physical limitations is required to apply scientific principles of conditioning and motivation techniques for establishing appropriate life-styles that include healthy exercise habits. In all appropriately supervised exercise sessions the goal should be to offer activities that will improve the participants' functional capacity. Exposure to and instruction in a variety of activities is encouraged. Positive attitudes toward work and play as well as positive physical benefits are desired outcomes.

Certain knowledge about leading physical activity for individuals can be learned. The instructor must be able to evaluate the physiologic effects of exercise and possess the ability to incorporate suitable and innovative activities for each individual. Preventive and rehabilitative programs require that participants not only establish, but adhere to, long-range commitments to regular physical activity in order to maintain optimal levels of fitness. Programs need to include motivational, counseling, teaching, and behavior modification techniques to emphasize current and valid health information and promote life-style changes. Knowledge of the scientific principles of exercise and conditioning, and the ability to design safe, appropriate, and enjoyable individualized exercise prescriptions, particularly for persons with cardiac disease, are the primary objectives for a well-prepared and competent exercise specialist.

Exercise Specialist

Behavioral Objectives. The exercise specialist, in addition to meeting the behavioral objectives outlined for the exercise test technologist, will demonstrate competence in exercise prescription and leadership in preventive and rehabilitative outpatient exercise programs for *participants with medically diagnosed disease or limitations, in particular, those with cardiac disease.*

1. *Exercise Prescription*
    GO The exercise specialist will demonstrate an understanding of the implications of exercise for persons with observed CHD risk factors and for patients with established cardiac, respiratory, metabolic, or orthopedic disorders and demonstrated competence in executing individualized exercise prescription.
    SLO Given sufficient medical information and the results of a graded exercise test or field tests, the exercise specialist will:
    A. Prior to the implementation of the exercise program use the test data for prescribing appropriate exercise, including intensity, duration, frequency, progression, type of physical activity, and whether exercise is to be supervised or unsupervised;
    B. Modify intensity and duration, temporarily or permanently, according to type of limitation (e.g., common metabolic, cardiorespiratory, and orthopedic);
    C. Demonstrate the use of a Goniometer and

describe exercise designed for improving mobility and flexibility of all major joints;

D. Demonstrate methods of determining percentage of body fat and specify normal measures based on sex and age;

E. Identify warm-up and cool-down phenomena with specific reference to angina and ischemic ECG changes;

F. Describe the inherent physiologic phenomena which exclude certain types of exercises from a rehabilitative exercise program;

G. Describe the physiologic consequences of certain postural changes, especially during the period following vigorous activity;

H. Describe exercises to improve strength, endurance, or flexibility in specific muscle groups;

I. Outline exercise programs of a continuous nature at a given intensity in contrast to programs of discontinuous exercise intensity (interval vs. continuous conditioning);

J. Demonstrate the most effective methods for accurate monitoring of exercise heart rate and physical effort;

K. Describe the precautions taken before, during, and after physical activity at high altitude and at different ambient temperatures and humidities with specific reference to the patient with cardiorespiratory limitations;

L. Describe contraindications to exercise or

inappropriate exercise responses which would be an indication for termination of the exercise session.

2. *Exercise Leadership*

GO The exercise specialist will demonstrate competence in leading physical activity in preventive and rehabilitative exercise programs.

SLO Given a case study and subject(s) lead appropriate exercises based on a prescription executed from the graded exercise test and other clinical and behavioral data.

SLO Describe common orthopedic problems associated with physical activity and adaptations required in the exercise prescription; include myositis ossificans, shin splints, tennis elbow, stress fracture, lordosis, and bone contusion of the os calcis.

SLO Explain a change in exercise prescription due to acute musculoskeletal problems, specifically bursitis, tendonitis, metatarsalgia, arthritis, and stone bruise.

GO The exercise specialist will demonstrate competence in the administrative concerns of effective exercise leadership.

A. Describe an organizational plan for facilities, equipment, and consumable supplies for an exercise program.

B. Describe considerations involved in scheduling events and staff.

C. Identify factors related to efficient data entry, storage, retrieval, and feedback to participants, physicians, and other involved persons.

    D. Implement evaluation procedures of testing, exercise, and patient education programs.

3. *Emergency Procedures*

  GO The exercise specialist will demonstrate competence in responding with the appropriate emergency procedures to situations which might arise prior, during, and after exercise.

  SLO Design and update emergency procedures for a preventive and rehabilitative exercise program.

4. *Functional Anatomy*

  GO The exercise specialist will demonstrate a knowledge of human functional anatomy.

  SLO Explain the properties and function of bone, muscle, and connective tissue.

  SLO Describe the functional anatomy of the cardiovascular and respiratory systems.

  SLO Given anatomic models, the exercise specialist will:

    A. Identify the major bones, muscle groups, and the diarthrodial joints of the human body; describe how each affects the joint range of motion;

    B. Identify the cardiovascular anatomy specifically, chambers, valves, vessels, and conduction system.

  SLO Describe differences in the mechanics of human locomotion in walking, jogging, running, and carrying or moving objects.

5. *Exercise Physiology*

GO The exercise specialist will demonstrate an understanding of exercise physiology.

SLO Diagram the cardiorespiratory system and list primary responses to increased energy demands during exercise.

SLO Describe the primary difference between aerobic and anaerobic metabolism and their relative importance in rehabilitative exercise programs.

SLO Define the properties of cardiac muscle, the generation of the action potential, and normal pathways of conduction.

SLO Describe the relationship between heart rate and blood pressure responses and aerobic capacity and adaptations to changing levels of chronic exercise in males and females of varying ages.

SLO Plot the following resting values and the normal response to increasing work intensity of heart rate (HR), stroke volume (SV), cardiac output ($\dot{Q}$), arteriovenous O_2 difference (a-vO_2 diff), O_2 uptake ($\dot{V}O_2$), systolic and diastolic blood pressure (SBP, DBP), minute ventilation ($\dot{V}_E$), tidal volume (TV), breathing frequency (f).

SLO Define and explain the concept of the Metabolic Equivalent Unit (MET) and kcal. Calculate the energy cost in METS and kcal for given exercise intensities in stepping exercise, bicycle ergometery, and during horizontal and grade walking and running.

SLO Explain the physiologic importance of the warm-up and cool-down, as specifically related to the cardiorespiratory system.

SLO Explain the difference in the cardiorespiratory responses to static (isometric) exercise compared with dynamic (isotonic) exercise; include possible hazards of isometric exercise for sedentary or symptomatic adults.

SLO Explain the specificity of conditioning and the physiologic differences among cardiorespiratory, endurance, and muscular strength conditioning; include the mechanism by which the functional capacity and hypertrophy increase during a conditioning program.

SLO Describe acceptable laboratory and field exercise test protocols from which functional capacity or $\dot{V}O_2$ max determinations or estimations may be obtained.

SLO Define the following terms: hyperphagia, dyspnea, hyperemia, ischemia, anemia, respiratory alkalosis and acidosis, angina pectoris, Valsalva maneuver, cardiac output, hypoxia, orthostatic hypotension, stroke volume, arterial pressures, calorimetry, hyperventilation, hyperpnea, hypoventilation.

6. *Pathophysiology*

GO The exercise specialist will demonstrate an understanding of the cardiorespiratory and metabolic responses to increasing intensities of exercise in certain diseases and conditions.

SLO Identify the cardiorespiratory and metabolic responses of myocardial dysfunction and ischemia at rest and during exercise.

SLO Identify the cardiorespiratory and metabolic responses of pulmonary disease at rest and during exercise.

SLO Identify the signs and symptoms of peripheral vascular diseases and the effects different kinds of exercise may have on each.

SLO Identify the metabolic responses and possible dysfunctions of a diabetic patient at rest and during exercise.

SLO Explain the influence of exercise on weight reduction and hyperlipidemia.

SLO Describe the effects of ambient temperature and humidity on functional capacity and the exercise prescription. Explain required adaptations to the exercise prescription when environmental extremes exist.

SLO List the principal effects of the action of the following classes of drugs (Appendix C).
   A. Antianginal
   B. Antiarrhythmic
   C. Anticoagulant
   D. Antiplatelet aggregation
   E. Antilipidemic
   F. Antihypertensive
   G. Digitalis glycosides

SLO List the major effects including ECG changes of the seven classes of drugs at rest and during exercise (Appendix D).

7. *Electrocardiography*

   GO The exercise specialist will demonstrate an understanding of the basic electrocardiographic responses at rest and during exercise.

   SLO Explain possible causes of ischemia and arrhythmias. Explain the significance of their occurrence during rest, exercise, and recovery.

   SLO Identify the potentially hazardous arrhythmias or conduction defects that might be observed on the ECG at rest or during exercise and explain what procedures would be followed concerning a participant's care.

   SLO Explain possible causes of ischemia and the significance of its occurrence during rest and exercise.

   SLO Identify the significance of the ECG abnormalities with special reference to exercise prescription and activity selection.

8. *Human Behavior/Psychology*

   GO The exercise specialist will demonstrate an understanding of basic behavioral psychology and group dynamics as they apply to exercise leadership.

   SLO Given a series of hypothetical situations involving participants in a preventive or rehabilitative exercise program, the exercise specialist will:

   A. Describe psychologic and physiologic responses to stressful situations. Discuss stress management techniques to elicit relaxation;

    B. Describe the appropriate motivational, counseling, and teaching techniques used in conducting exercise and promoting life-style changes;

    C. Define or describe each of the following terms in relation to the management of an exercise program: aggression, hostility, projection, denial, play, identification, hedonism, goal orientation and setting, operant conditioning, rapport, recreation, anxiety, empathy, fear, rationalization, relaxation, opinions-attitudes motivation, euphoria, depression, rejection, and catharsis.

9. *Gerontology*

GO The exercise specialist will demonstrate an understanding of the special problems of the older participant.

SLO List the differences in conditioning older vs. younger participants.

SLO Identify common orthopedic problems of older participants and explain modifications of exercise to avoid aggravation of the disabilities.

SLO Describe leadership techniques which might need to be adjusted because of vision or hearing impairments of participants.

10. *Internship*

In order to add to the theoretical knowledge and abilities required for an exercise specialist in leading either individual or group exercise programs, an internship of at least 6 months (800 hours) is required. This internship should occur under the direction of a certified program director or physician who has a leadership role in preventive or rehabilitative testing and exercise programs for *participants with medically diagnosed disease or limitations, particularly cardiac disease.*

The internship should include a variety of experiences, such as graded exercise testing, exercise prescription, supervision of the individual exercise programs, and leading group exercises. These exercise programs should include participants with medical or physical limitations, specifically cardiorespiratory disease.

Evaluation of the exercise leader will involve a written and oral examination in the above content areas (1 to 10) as well as a practical demonstration of leading an exercise session. The following characteristics must be demonstrated for competency:

A. Adequate organization of a session into warm-up, endurance (aerobic) activity, and cool-down periods;

B. Maintaining individual adherence to the exercise prescription;

C. Ability to present a variety of activities;

D. Ability to make quick modifications (individually or for the group) based on observations during an exercise session;

E. Ability to create a relaxed and enjoyable "atmosphere" among the participants;

F. Ability to demonstrate competent emergency procedures.

C. PREVENTIVE AND REHABILITATIVE EXERCISE PROGRAM DIRECTOR

Exercise appears to have an appropriate and accepted role in both preventive and rehabilitative medical programs. As a result, there is an increasing demand for information about exercise testing, exercise prescription, and exercise programs by the medical and health-related professions and by the general public. In order to meet this demand an increasing number of qualified, specially trained exercise program directors are needed.

Because the persons who wish to become exercise program directors must have the knowledge and competencies of the exercise test technologist and exercise specialist, it is probable that they have already had much of the practical background necessary for the testing and physical conditioning portions of the program. To understand the medical and physiologic implications of graded exercise testing and the resulting exercise programs and to understand how and why certain activities are recommended or contraindicated, more theoretical experience is needed. It is hoped that the majority of this knowledge will have been obtained during studies for an advanced degree in fields such as exercise physiology, physiology and medicine, or physical education.

Since the exercise program directors are responsible for (1) the inclusion of adequate exercise testing procedures, (2) accurate, individualized exercise prescription, and (3) careful supervision and leadership of a safe, effective, and enjoyable exercise program, they need the theoretical and practical backgrounds associated with certain aspects of medicine, physiology, physical education, and behavioral psychology. Thus, exercise program directors are unique specialists in that they must draw from a wide range of abilities, knowledge, and experience as they relate to exercise.

With this combination of theoretical knowledge and practical experience, the exercise program director should be capable of organizing and administering all types of programs in any situation. The exercise program director should have the ability to plan and initiate new programs, as well as to reorganize and upgrade existing ones. The fact that one can work in programs for disease-limited patients and asymptomatic persons suggests that they possess the versatility, adaptability, and breadth of knowledge and experience necessary for certification as a preventive and rehabilitative exercise program director. The same may not be the case for those who have worked only with athletes or children. It is for this reason that there is so much emphasis on the preventive and rehabilitative aspects of exercise.

The exact role of the exercise program director depends on factors such as personal interest, the size of the program, and the type of people who will be tested and exercised. If the program is small, then the exercise program director may be involved in the collection and analysis of data obtained during exercise testing or the supervision and leadership of the actual exercise programs. If the program is relatively large, then the duties may be primarily administrative and related to the actual prescription of the activity program in close cooperation with the physician. The exercise program director's duties will also include the training, continuing education, and supervision of the other personnel, i.e., the exercise test technologists and exercise specialists. The exercise program director should understand the basic aspects of the physiology of exercise and training, psychologic aspects of behavior modification, emergency procedures, and particular problems of special groups of patients.

An exercise program director must also work with and communicate with the public, those persons who are tested and who are exercised, and with physicians and health professionals, i.e., with people who have varying degrees of knowledge and sophistication regarding the medical, physiologic, psychologic, and educational aspects of exercise programs. Because of this, the exercise program director should understand and be able to explain and discuss both the theoretical and practical aspects of exercise and conditioning with each of these various groups of people. This ability to communicate is especially important since people in exercise programs should be able not only to improve their physical condition, but also to acquire a certain degree of autonomy in that improvement. For example, participants cannot always remain in a supervised, controlled exercise program. For this reason, a program of continuing education is important so that the participants can continue to lead active, more healthful lives when they no longer desire or are not able to continue in a program.

In special programs for middle-aged or older persons, for persons who have a high risk of developing a disease such as coronary heart disease, or for those who already have specific medical problems, the exercise program director must understand the medical and physiologic implications of the medical history of these patients and provide for any special needs related to the testing, prescription, and supervision of exercises. In doing this, the exercise program director is expected to maintain a close working relationship with appropriate medical specialists. In such cases where the knowledge and experience necessary to work with these special groups are inadequate and were not integral parts of their educational background, exercise program directors are expected to study and learn more about any special aspects of a particular medical or physiologic problem by means of special courses or symposia, by reading scientific articles and books, by discussions with knowledgeable persons, and by conducting research. In other words, exercise program directors should be "life-time students" who continually strive to improve the level of competency within their specialty.

Professional study and cooperation of the exercise program director with physicians, physiologists, physical educators, and other health personnel are basic to the optimal realization of health benefits from physical activity programs. This type of team work is especially needed if the benefits from these programs are to be made available to large segments of the public. The exercise program director can and should be a major factor in the success of such a program.

Exercise Program Director

Behavioral Objectives. The exercise program director, in addition to meeting the behavioral objectives outlined for the exercise specialist and exercise test technologist, will demonstrate competency in designing, implementing, and administering preventive and rehabilitative exercise programs and educating the staff and members of the community about physical activity in programs of disease prevention and rehabilitation. This includes the following behavioral objectives.

1. *Program Administration*

   GO The exercise program director will understand the role of administration as a means of program facilitation.

   SLO Diagram and explain an organizational chart and show the staff relationships between an exercise program director, governing body, exercise specialist, exercise test technologist, medical advisor, participant's personal physician, and participants.

   SLO Identify and explain operating policies for preventive and rehabilitative exercise programs including data analysis and reporting, confidentiality of records, relationships between program and referring physicians, continuing education of staff, continuing education of participant and family, legal liability, accident or injury reporting, emergency procedures, and hiring and firing.

   SLO Explain the legal concepts of tort, negligence, contributory negligence, liability, standards of care, consent, contract, confidentiality, and malpractice.

   SLO Describe and explain program evaluation.

   SLO Design physical facilities necessary for exercise programs.

SLO Identify safety requirements and equipment.

SLO Explain concepts of budget development.

SLO Describe and explain strategies of public and human relations, including techniques for informing members of the community about physical activity programs of prevention and rehabilitation.

SLO Design and coordinate research efforts which may evolve from testing, exercise, or educational programs.

SLO Interpret applied research in the areas of testing, exercise, and educational programs in order to update programs and stay current with the state-of-the-art.

2. *Emergency Procedures*

GO The exercise program director will demonstrate competence in the use, maintenance, and updating of appropriate emergency equipment, supplies, and evacuation plans.

SLO Teach the principles and techniques used in cardiopulmonary resuscitation.

SLO Demonstrate the emergency procedures, equipment, and materials needed during testing and exercise sessions.

SLO Discuss the individual responsibility and legal implications related to emergency care.

3. *Functional Anatomy*

GO The program director will demonstrate knowledge of human functional anatomy.

SLO Explain how the human mechanism influences performance with implications for the selection and conduct of physical exercise.

SLO Analyze and evaluate varieties of exercises and movements to predict their influence upon structure, growth, efficiency, and health.

4. *Exercise Physiology*
   GO The exercise program director will demonstrate a knowledge and a theoretical understanding of exercise physiology.
   SLO Demonstrate an understanding of the basic electrophysiology of cardiac muscle by explaining the properties of cardiac muscle and the normal and abnormal conduction patterns of the propagation of action potentials across the myocardium.
   SLO Demonstrate an understanding of the relationship between muscle structure and function.
   A. Describe the structure of muscle fiber.
   B. Describe functional characteristics of histochemical classifications of skeletal muscle fibers.
   C. Explain contraction of muscle in terms of the sliding filament theory.
   D. Explain twitch, summation, and tetanus in terms of muscle contraction.
   E. Explain the biochemistry of muscle fatigue under specific conditions of task, intensity, and duration of exercise.
   SLO Demonstrate an understanding of the metabolic and cardiorespiratory response to exercise and explain their interrelationships.
   A. Describe and explain the mechanisms by which heart rate (HR), stroke volume

(SV), cardiac output ($\dot{Q}$), arteriovenous O_2 difference (a-vO_2 diff), O_2 uptake ($\dot{V}O_2$), systolic, diastolic blood pressure (SBP, DBP), minute ventilation ($\dot{V}_E$), tidal volume (TV), breathing frequency (f), and respiratory quotient (RQ), change with increasing work intensities in conditioned and unconditioned adults of varying ages (some physiologic mechanisms may not be known).

B. Describe the physiologic changes which would lower myocardial oxygen consumption for a given submaximal exercise intensity following a physical conditioning program.

C. Explain the contribution of aerobic and anaerobic metabolism to the total energy cost of exercise at maximum and at different intensities of exercise.

D. Describe the biochemistry of muscle fatigue under specific conditions of task, intensity, and duration of exercise.

E. Explain the adaptations and characteristics which differentiate the conditioned from the unconditioned adult, in particular cardiorespiratory and musculoskeletal changes.

F. Explain the concept of the reversibility of conditioning.

5. *Pathophysiology*

GO The exercise program director will understand the interrelationship between different diseases or conditions and physical activity.

SLO Explain the process of atherosclerosis.

SLO Explain the causes and mechanisms of myocardial ischemia and infarction.

SLO Explain the causes and mechanisms of hypertension, obesity, diabetes, arthritis, gout, and of pulmonary disease.

SLO Identify and explain the effects of the above diseases or conditions on cardiorespiratory and metabolic function at rest and during exercise.

SLO Explain the risk factor concept of CHD and the influence of heredity and life-style upon the development of CHD.

SLO Explain the diagnostic and prognostic value of the results of the graded exercise test.

SLO Identify and explain the mechanisms by which exercise may contribute to preventing the above diseases and rehabilitating individuals with the above diseases.

SLO Describe muscular, cardiorespiratory, and metabolic responses to exercise following a decrease in physical activity, bed rest, or casting of a limb for a period of 1 month.

SLO Name at least one drug from each of the following classes, explain the mechanism of its principal action, and list its major side-effects, including ECG changes at rest and during exercise (Appendix C–D).

    A. Antianginal

    B. Antiarrhythmic

    C. Anticoagulant

    D. Antiplatelet aggregation

    E. Antilipidemic

    F. Antihypertensive
    G. Digitalis glycosides
    H. Other agents
    I. Bronchodilators
    J. Hypoglycemics
    K. ''Mood'' elevators; stimulants

6. *Electrocardiography*

    GO The program director will understand electrocardiographic responses at rest and during exercise testing and conditioning.

    SLO Identify ECG evidence of myocardial infarction and explain the significance of the changes seen on the ECG.

    SLO Explain the diagnostic and prognostic value of occurrence of ischemic or arrhythmic responses at rest, during exercise, and at recovery.

    SLO Explain possible causes of a false positive or false negative exercise test. Discuss methods of avoiding a false positive/negative exercise test.

    SLO Explain the functioning of cardiac pacemakers and the precautions to be taken by individuals with pacemakers.

7. *Human Behavior/Psychology*

    GO The exercise program director will demonstrate an understanding of basic principles of human behavior and group dynamics to include communication, motivation, and factors which influence behavior over time.

    SLO Identify and explain factors supporting or inhibiting behavior changes such as initiating an exercise program.

SLO Establish means of assessing the factors supporting or inhibiting behavior changes.

SLO Identify and explain factors influencing the effectiveness of communication.

GO The exercise program director will demonstrate an understanding of the effect of psychologic stress on physiologic processes.

SLO Identify physiologic mechanisms by which stress may produce undesirable effects.

8. *Gerontology*

GO The exercise program director will demonstrate an understanding of the effect of the aging process on the structure and function of the human organism at rest, during exercise, and after conditioning.

SLO Identify and explain the cardiorespiratory response to exercise in persons of advancing age.

SLO Explain the differences in conditioning of older compared to younger participants, with regard to strength, functional capacity, mechanical efficiency, reaction and movement time, flexibility, coordination, and tolerance to heat and cold.

SLO Describe common orthopedic problems of older participants and explain how modifications of exercise can reduce their aggravation.

9. *Internship*

In order to qualify as an exercise program director, an internship or period of practical experience of at least 1 year is required. The internship should be under the supervision of a certified exercise program director and a physician and provide opportunities to obtain competencies in administration, program leadership, laboratory procedures, and exercise prescription. It is assumed that the preceptor of the internship will work closely with the prospective exercise program director. In addition to the opportunity to demonstrate proficiency, oral and written examinations are an integral part of the learning experience.

Appendix A

Informed Consent for Graded Exercise Test*

1. *Explanation of the Graded Exercise Test*

   You will perform a graded exercise test on a bicycle ergometer or a motor-driven treadmill. The exercise intensities will begin at a level you can easily accomplish and will be advanced in stages, depending on your functional capacity. We may stop the test at any time because of signs of fatigue or you may stop when you wish to because of personal feelings of fatigue or discomfort. We do not wish you to exercise at a level which is abnormally uncomfortable for you; however, for maximum benefit from the test, exercise as long as is comfortable.

2. *Risks and Discomforts*

   There exists the possibility of certain changes occurring during the test. They include abnormal blood pressure, fainting, disorders of heart beat, and in rare instances, heart attack. Every effort will be made to minimize these through the preliminary examination and by observations during testing. Emergency equipment and trained personnel are

---

*When test is for a purpose other than diagnosis or prescription, e.g., experimental interest, this should be indicated on the Informed Consent Form.

available to deal with unusual situations which may arise.

3. *Benefits to be Expected*

The results obtained from the exercise test may assist in the diagnosis of your illness or in evaluating in what types of physical activities you might engage with no or low hazards.

4. *Inquiries*

Any question about the procedures used in the graded exercise test or in the estimation of functional capacity are encouraged. If you have any doubts or questions, please ask us for further explanations.

5. *Freedom of Consent*

Your permission to perform this graded exercise test is voluntary. You are free to deny consent if you so desire.

I have read this form and I understand the test procedures that I will perform. I consent to participate in this test.

_____

Signature of Patient

_____   _____

Date   Witness

Questions: _____

_____

Response: _____

Physician signature: optional.

*Policy on Human Subjects for Research is available on request from ACSM.

Medical Referral Form for Participation in Graded Exercise Testing and Exercise Program

Your patient _____ has applied to participate in the _____ exercise program. This program will require your patient to participate in a graded exercise test and exercise classes. Active participation in the program requires your medical clearance. Please complete the following form if there are no contraindications for participation in the program.

Patient: _____ Date: _____

Address: _____

Telephone Number: _____ Date of Birth: _____ Sex: _____

Basis of Referral: _____ Diagnostic Screening for CHD _____ Functional Capacity _____ Exercise Prescription
_____ Improvement Assessment

1. Present Coronary Artery Disease Status:
   _____ Yes _____ No   A.   Normal
   _____ Yes _____ No   B.   Coronary Prone (3 CHD Risk Factors)
   _____ Yes _____ No   C.   Post MI
   Number Documented Infarctions   1   2   3   4   (Please circle)
   Time Since First MI: _____ Months   Time Since Last MI: _____ Months
   Complications of any infarction: _____ Congestive Failure   _____ Cardiogenic Shock
                                        _____ Serious Arrhythmia   _____ Post Infarction Angina

Yes _____ No _____ D. Post Coronary Artery Bypass Surgery

Yes _____ No _____ E. Post Valve or Open Heart Surgery

F. Angina

Yes _____ No _____ Typical Angina

Yes _____ No _____ Atypical Angina

Time Since First Angina: _____ Months

Angina Related to: _____ Effort _____ Rest (Awake) _____ Emotion _____ Nocturnal

Present Trend of Angina: _____ Decreasing _____ Increasing _____ Stable _____ On Therapy

Yes _____ No _____ G. Arrhythmias

_____ ≤6 PVC/min _____ >6 PVC/min _____ Multifocal or Multiform PVC

_____ Ventricular Tachycardia _____ Idioventricular _____ Couplets

_____ Supraventricular Tachycardia

_____ Atrial Fibrillation _____ Junctional _____ Atrial Flutter _____ Atrial Tachycardia

_____ Sinus Bradycardia

_____ Other

2. Associated Medical Conditions:

Yes _____ No _____ Congenital Heart Defect

Yes _____ No _____ Peripheral Vascular (claudication)

Yes _____ No _____ Valvular Heart Disease

_____ AS _____ AR _____ MS _____ MR

Yes _____ No _____ Hyperuricemia

Yes _____ No _____ COPD

Yes _____ No _____ Diabetes

Yes _____ No _____ Hyperlipidemia

_____ TYPE I _____ TYPE II

_____ TYPE III _____ TYPE IV

_____ Triglycerides _____ HDL

Yes _____ No _____ Systemic Hypertension _____ Cholesterol

Yes _____ No _____ Family History of CAD _____ Presently a Smoker

Amount/day _____

Orthopedic Limitations (Specify) _____

Neurologic Limitations (Specify) _____

Allergies (Specify) _____

3. Prior Cardiac Operation

		Date	Hospital
Yes ___ No ___	Coronary Artery Bypass Graft	_____	_____
Yes ___ No ___	IMA Bypass Graft/Implant	_____	_____
Yes ___ No ___	Peripheral Bypass Graft	_____	_____
Yes ___ No ___	Aortic Valve Operation	_____	_____
Yes ___ No ___	Aortic Valve Replacement	_____	_____
Yes ___ No ___	Aneurysmectomy	_____	_____
Yes ___ No ___	VDS Repair Post Infarct	_____	_____

Other (Specify) _____

4. Current Medications and Dosage

Medication	Dosage mg/day	Type
_____	_____	_____
_____	_____	_____
_____	_____	_____
_____	_____	_____

5. Physical Examination:
   A. Blood Pressure   Supine ___ RA ___ LA   Standing ___ RA ___ LA
   B. Heart Rate   Supine ___   Standing ___
   C. Heart Sounds
      Normal S₂ ___ Yes ___ No
      Gallop Rhythm
         S₃ ___ Yes ___ No   Thrills ___ Yes ___ No
         S₄ ___ Yes ___ No   Sustained LV Impulse ___ Yes ___ No
   D. Cardiac Murmur ___ Yes ___ No
      Systolic ___ Early ___ Mid ___ Late   Systolic Click ___ Yes ___ No
      Diastolic ___ Early ___ Mid ___ Late
      Grade (I–VI) ___

E. Bruits

Right Carotid _____ Yes _____ No
Left Carotid _____ Yes _____ No
Abdominal Aorta _____ Yes _____ No
Groin _____ Yes _____ No

F. Pulses

Carotid	_____ Normal	_____ Decreased	_____ Absent
Axillary	_____ Normal	_____ Decreased	_____ Absent
Brachial	_____ Normal	_____ Decreased	_____ Absent
Radial	_____ Normal	_____ Decreased	_____ Absent
Ulnar	_____ Normal	_____ Decreased	_____ Absent
Abdominal Aorta	_____ Normal	_____ Decreased	_____ Absent
Femoral	_____ Normal	_____ Decreased	_____ Absent
Popliteal	_____ Normal	_____ Decreased	_____ Absent
Post Tibial	_____ Normal	_____ Decreased	_____ Absent
Dorsalis Pedis	_____ Normal	_____ Decreased	_____ Absent

G. Evidence of Chronic Lung Disease _____ Yes _____ No

Chest Deformity _____ Yes _____ No
Scoliosis _____ Yes _____ No
Rales, Wheezes _____ Yes _____ No
Hepatomegaly _____ Yes _____ No
Edema _____ Yes _____ No

Bone or Joint Abnormalities _____ Yes _____ No
(Specify) _____

Neurological _____
(Specify) _____

H. Xanthoma _____ Yes _____ No
Arcus Lipoides _____ Yes _____ No
Bilateral Earlobe Creases _____ Yes _____ No
High Arch Palate _____ Yes _____ No
Palpable Thyroid _____ Yes _____ No

122

I. Laboratory Findings
   Blood Hemoglobin —— Hematocrit —— White Blood Cell ——
6. 12 Lead ECG Interpretation (Please enclose)

Indicate Site of Change

	Yes	No	Anterolateral I,AVL,V_4-V_6	Anteroseptal V_1-V_3	Anteroapical V_3-V_4	Posterior V_1	Posterolateral V_4-V_6	Inferior II,III,AVF	Inferolateral II,III,AVF, V_4-V_6
Infarction (Q-Pattern)									
ST-Junctional Segment Depression									
T-Wave Abnormality									
ST-Segment Elevation									

123

_____ Yes _____ No QRS Axis Deviation
       _____ Left _____ Right _____ Extreme _____ Indeterminate

_____ Yes _____ No Ventricular Hypertrophy (High Amplitude R-Waves)
       _____ LVH _____ RVH

_____ Yes _____ No Atrioventricular Conduction Defect
       _____ Complete (3°) _____ Partial (2°) _____ P–R _____ 0.22 sec (1°)
       _____ WPW _____ Short R–R _____ Pacemaker

_____ Yes _____ No Ventricular Conduction Defect
       _____ RBBB _____ LBBB _____ LAH _____ LVH Other: _____

_____ Yes _____ No Low-Amplitude QRS Transition Zone
       _____ V_2 _____ V_3 _____ V_4 _____ V_5 _____ V_6

7. Indicate if previously performed and enclose copy of report if available
 _____ Yes _____ No Graded Exercise Test _____ With Thallium _____ Without Thallium
 _____ Yes _____ No Coronary Arteriogram or Other Angiography
 _____ Yes _____ No Radionuclide Ventriculogram
       Type of Study Performed _____
 _____ Yes _____ No Echocardiogram

I know of no reason why my patient _____ should not be able to
undertake a graded exercise test and participate in a cardiac rehabilitation program.

Physician's Signature _____ Date _____
Address _____ Phone _____

124

Appendix C

Pharmacologic Agents Which May Be Encountered in Cardiac Patients

(The list of named drugs is neither inclusive nor exhaustive)

I. Antianginal Agents
  A. Nitrates: nitroglycerin (NITRO-BID), isosorbide dinitrate (ISORDIL, SORBITRATE, ISORDIL TEMBIDS), erythrityl tetranitrate (CARDILATE), pentaerythritol tetranitrate (PERITRATE), ethaverine-pentaerythritol tetranitrate (PAPAVATRAL)
  B. Beta-blocking agents: propranolol hydrochloride (INDERAL), metoprolol tartrate (LOPRESSOR)
  C. Alpha-blocking agents: phentolamine (REGITINE)
II. Antiarrhythmic Agents
  A. Digoxin (LANOXIN), diphenylhydantoin (DILANTIN), lidocaine (XYLOCAINE), procainamide hydrochloride (PRONESTYL), propranolol hydrochloride (INDERAL), metoprolol tartrate (LOPRESSOR), quinidine gluconate (QUINAGLUTE DURA-TABS), quinidine sulfate (QUINIDEX EXTENTABS), quinidine polygalacturonate (CARDIOQUIN).

III. Anticoagulant Agents
  A. Sodium heparin (HEPATHROM, LIPO-HEPIN, LIQUMAEIN SODIUM), bishydroxycoumarin (DICUMAROL), sodium warfarin (COUMADIN)
IV. Antiplatelet Aggregation Agents
  A. Sulfinpyrazone (ANTURANE)
  B. Acetyl salicylic acid (ASPIRIN)
IV. Antilipid Agents
  A. Clofibrate (ATROMID-S), cholestyramine (CUEMID, QUESTRAN), nicotinic acid (NIACIN)
VI. Antihypertensive Agents
  A. Diuretics:
    (1) benzothiadiazines: chlorothiazide (DIURIL), hydrochlorothiazide (ESIDRIX, HYDRODIURIL), methyclothiazide (ENDURON)
    (2) Loop diuretics: furosemide (LASIX), ethacrynic acid (EDECRIN)
    (3) potassium sparing: spironolactone (ALDACTONE), triamterene, (DYRENIUM)
  B. Vasodilator:
    (1) hydralazine (APRESOLINE)
    (2) prazosin hydrochloride (MINIPRESS)
  C. Drugs affecting sympathetic nervous system:
    (1) reserpine (SERPASIL), guanethidine sulfate (ISMELIN), propranolol (INDERAL), metoprolol (LOPRESSOR) alpha-methyldopa (ALDOMET), clonidine (CATAPRES), prazosin (MINIPRESS)

D. Others: spironolactone-hydrochlorothiazide (ALDACTAZIDE), methyldopa-hydrochlorothiazide (ALDORIL), chlorothiazide-reserpine (DIUPRES), chlorthalidone-reserpine (REGROTON), chlorthalidone (HYGROTON), acetazolamide (DIAMOX), dyrenium-hydrochlorothiazide (DYAZIDE)

VII. Digitalis Glycoside Agents
   A. ouabain (STROPHANTHIN-G), digitoxin (CRYSTODIGIN), digoxin (LANOXIN)

VIII. OTHER AGENTS:
   A. Bronchodilators: (ISUPREL, BRONKO-TABS, QUADRINAL, TEDRAL, VERE-QUAD)
   B. Major Tranquilizers: phenothiazines (THORAZINE, MELLARIL, COM-PAZINE)
   C. Tricyclic Antidepressants: (TOFRANIL, ELAVIL, NORPRAMIN)
   D. Antianxiety Agents: meprobamate (MIL-TOWN, EQUANIL), chlordiazepoxide (LIBRIUM), diazepam (VALIUM)
   E. LITHIUM CARBONATE
   F. Thyroid: SYNTHROID, THYROID USP
   G. Antihistamines
   H. Hypoglycemic agents—oral or insulin
   I. Alcohol
   J. Nicotine
   K. Estrogens

Appendix D

Cardiac and Noncardiac Drug Interventions and Their Possible Effect on Exercise Regimens

(The list of named drugs is neither inclusive nor exhaustive)

Certified staff should be aware of the following information about each participant prior to beginning a graded test or exercise session.

1. All drugs taken by each participant.
2. The medical indications for each drug.
3. The pharmacodynamics and pharmacokinetics of each drug.

		Effect			
	Exercise Performance	Heart Rate	Blood Pressure	Effect on ECG	Effect on GXT
Antianginal Nitrates/Agents	↑ Nitrobid ↑ Isordil ↑ Isordic Tembids ↑ Cardilate ↑ Peritrate	↑ Nitrobid ↑ Sorbitrate ↑ Ointment	↓ Nitrobid ↓ Sorbitrate ↓ Ointment	Reduces evidence of myocardial ischemia	May delay onset of "ischemic response" (lower double product)
Beta Blockers	↕ Inderal ↕ Lopressor	↓ Inderal ↓ Lopressor	↓ Inderal ↓ Lopressor	U waves may become prominent due to bradycardia	May delay onset of "ischemic response" (lower double product)
Antihypertensive Diuretics		→ Diuril, Esidrix → Enduron, Lasix → Edecrin, Aldactone → Dyrenium	↓ Diuril, Esidrix ↓ Enduron, Lasix ↓ Edecrin, ↓ Aldactone ↓ Dyrenium	Prolongs QT interval, accentuates U waves if hypokalemic	May cause False-Positive if hypokalemic
Vasodilator		↑ Apresoline	↓ Apresoline		
Central Nervous System		↓ Serpasil ↓ Ismelin ↓ Inderal	↓ Serpasil ↓ Ismelin ↓ Inderal, Minipress ↓ Aldomet, Catapres		May delay onset of "ischemic response"
Digitalis Glycosides	↑ Strophanthin-G ↑ Crystodigin ↑ Lanoxin	↑ With toxicity or may ↓ if Blocks A–V node		May produce S–T depression or sagging change accentuated with exercise	False-Positive

Antiarrhythmics	↑ Lanoxin ↑ Dilantin ↕ Xylocaine ↑ Pronestyl ↕ Inderal ↕ Lopressor ↕ Quinaglute	↑ Pronestyl ↑ Quinaglute ↑ Norpace	No change	ST–T wave changes, U-wave changes, widening of QRS, QT changes	Lanoxin—False-Positive Quinaglute, Inderal—may delay onset of "ischemic response"
Tranquilizers (phenothiazines)		↑	→	T&U wave changes	May cause False-Positive
Antidepressants	Minor Antiarrythmics Effect	↑	→	ST–T wave changes	May cause False-Positive
Antianxiety (lithium)	No change	No change	No change	ST–T wave changes	May cause False-Positive
Others Nicotine Bronchodilators Antihistamines with Decon- gestants Thyroid Drugs Cold Remedies Alcohol		↑ ↓ ↓ ↓ ↓	↑ ↓ ↓ ↓ ↓ →	 No change No change No change ? ?	May cause False-Positive ? No change No change ? ?

Appendix E

Informed Consent For Cardiac Out-Patient Rehabilitation Program

1. Explanation of Out-Patient Cardiac Rehabilitation Program

You will be placed on a rehabilitation program that will include physical exercises. The levels of exercise which you will undertake will be based on your cardiovascular response to an initial graded exercise test. You will be given explicit instructions regarding the amount and kind of regular exercise you should do. Organized exercise sessions will be available on a regularly scheduled basis. Your exercise sessions may be adjusted by the exercise specialist in consultation with the exercise program director and physician depending on your progress. You will be given the opportunity for re-evaluation with a graded exercise test _____ months after the initiation of the rehabilitation program, and _____ thereafter. Other retests may be recommended as needed.

2. Monitoring

Your pre-exercise blood pressure will be monitored as required. You will monitor your own pulse rate before, during, and after each exercise session. In addition, ECG monitoring of your exercise prescription will be performed on a _____ basis or as needed.

3. Risks and Discomforts

There exists the possibility of certain changes occurring during the exercise sessions. These include abnormal blood pressure, fainting, disorders of heart beat, and in rare instances heart attack. Every effort will be made to minimize them by the preliminary examination and by observations during exercise. Emergency equipment and trained personnel are available to deal with unusual situations which may arise.

4. Benefits to be Expected

Participation in the rehabilitation program may not benefit you directly in any way. The results obtained may help in evaluating in what types of activities you might engage safely in your daily life. No assurance can be given that the rehabilitation program will increase your functional capacity although widespread experience indicates that improvement is usually achieved.

5. Responsibility of the Participant

To gain expected benefits you must give priority to *regular attendance* and adherence to prescribed amounts of intensity, duration, frequency, progression, and *type of activity*.

To achieve the best possible *preventive* health care:

DO *NOT*: A. Withhold any information pertinent to symptoms from the exercise specialist, nurse, physician, exercise program director, or other professional personnel.

B. Exceed target heart rate.

C. Exercise when you do not feel well.

D. Exercise within 2 hours after eating.

E. Exercise after drinking alcoholic beverages.

F. Use extremely hot shower after exercising (stay out of sauna, steam bath, and similar extreme temperatures).

G. Undertake isometric or straining exercises.

DO:

A. Report any unusual symptom which you experience before, during, or after exercise, or you notice in an exercising colleague.

B. Check in with the exercise specialist after showering/dressing before leaving the site. If you plan to use other facilities at the site, please indicate that you will be doing so to the exercise specialist. At that time you must accept responsibility for yourself, and exercise *at your own risk*.

6. Use of Medical Records

The information which is obtained during exercise testing and while I am a participant in the Cardiac Rehabilitation program will be treated as privileged and confidential. It is not to be released or revealed to any person except my referring physician without my written consent. The information obtained however, may be used for statistical analysis or scientific purpose with my right to privacy retained.

7. Inquiries

Any questions about the rehabilitation program are welcome. If you have doubts or questions, please ask us for further explanation.

8. Freedom of Consent

Your permission to engage in this Rehabilitation Program is voluntary. You are free to deny consent if you so desire, both now and at any point in the program.

I acknowledge that I have read this form in its entirety or it has been read to me and that I understand the Rehabilitation Program in which I will be engaged. I accept the rules and regulations set forth. I consent to participate in this Rehabilitation Program.

Questions: _____

_____

_____

Response: _____

_____

_____

_____

Signature of Patient

_____

Date

_____

Witness

Appendix F

Calculation of the Energy Requirements in METS for Various Activities

There is a need for a simple means for describing the energy requirements of steady-state exercise. Use of the number of multiples of the resting metabolic rate (METS) serves this purpose. One MET is the equivalent of the resting oxygen consumption ($\dot{V}O_2$) which is approximately 3.5 ml/kg·min (1 MET = 3.5 ml/kg·min). The MET level during exercise is determined by dividing the exercise metabolic rate, represented by the exercise $\dot{V}O_2$, by the resting metabolic rate, represented by the resting $\dot{V}O_2$. Since measurement of oxygen consumption during exercise is not always possible, estimates of MET equivalents for certain activities can be made using the information that follows.

The exercise staff should be familiar with equations for the calculation of the energy requirements of several basic physical activities, e.g. walking, running, stepping, and cycling. Once the mechanics of calculation are learned, the exercise staff may use the relationships to prepare the exercise prescription and to determine relative energy expenditure in METS for various physical activities. For ease of understanding, the respective calculations are set forth as a series of arithmetic and algebraic steps.

The energy requirements for horizontal walking and running can be estimated with a reasonable degree of accuracy for walking speeds from 50 to 100 m/min (1.9 to 3.7 mph) and for running speeds exceeding 134 m/min (5.0 mph). Relatively accurate estimates are more difficult to obtain for speeds between 100 m/min and 134 m/min because walking and running patterns in this range vary greatly among individuals, mainly because of differences in body size or leg length. The energy requirement for walking increases linearly and predictably for speeds between 50 and 100 m/min, and exponentially thereafter. The energy requirement for running increases in a linear and predictable manner for speeds greater than 134 m/min. Below 134 m/min there is a "gray area" between fast walking and slow jogging that makes it nearly impossible to predict the energy costs with any degree of accuracy.

Walking

A. Estimation of the energy requirements for *horizontal* walking.

$\dot{V}O_2$ in ml/kg·min = speed in m/min × 0.1 ml O_2/kg·min per m/min × kg body wt + 1 MET or 3.5 ml/kg·min ÷ kg body wt

Multiply by body weight in kg to obtain the rate of total oxygen uptake ($\dot{V}O_2$). Divide by body weight (kg) to express the $\dot{V}O_2$ in ml/kg·min. These two body weights cancel and the formula is reduced to:

$\dot{V}O_2$ in ml/kg·min = speed in m/min × 0.1 ml O_2/kg·min per m/min* + 3.5 ml O_2/kg·min.

*The energy requirement for walking one meter/min = 0.1 ml/kg·min per m/min.

EXAMPLE:

Question: What values for $\dot{V}O_2$ and METS correspond to a horizontal walking speed of 80 m/min (3 mph or 4.8 km/hr)?

$\dot{V}O_2$ = 80 m/min × 0.1 ml/kg·min per m/min + 3.5 ml/kg·min = 11.5 ml/kg·min

METS = 11.5 ml/kg·min ÷ 3.5 ml/kg·min = 3.3

Question: A cardiac patient must exercise at a $\dot{V}O_2$ of 13.2 ml/kg·min (3.7 METS). What speed do you set on the horizontal treadmill to achieve this value?

Answer: 13.2 ml/kg·min = ? m/min × 0.1 ml/kg·min per m/min + 3.5 ml/kg·min

Subtract one MET from total exercise $\dot{V}O_2$ to obtain *NET* $\dot{V}O_2$ for walking.

13.2 ml/kg·min − 3.5 ml/kg·min = 9.7 ml/kg·min = NET $\dot{V}O_2$

Divide the NET $\dot{V}O_2$ by the net energy requirement for walking one meter/min = (0.1 ml/kg·min per m/min). The units cancel and the answer is 97 m/min.

$$\frac{9.7 \text{ ml}}{\text{kg·min}} \div \frac{0.1 \text{ ml}}{\text{kg·min}} \times \frac{\text{min}}{\text{m}} = 97 \text{ m/min or}$$

$$\frac{97 \text{ m/min}}{26.8 \text{ m/min}} = 3.6 \text{ mph}$$

(1 mph = 26.8 m/min = 1.6 km/hr).

B. Grade walking at speeds between 50 and 100 m/min. This calculation is divided into two parts:

    1. The horizontal speed component is calculated as in A, above.

    2. The vertical work component makes use of

the relationship: 1 kilogram meter (kgm) of work requires 1.8 ml of oxygen. In addition vertical work equals per cent grade × walking speed in m/min × kg body weight. The resulting answer is divided by kg body weight so that the value is expressed in ml of oxygen per kilogram (kg) of body weight. Thus, the body weight (kg) used to calculate vertical work will cancel with body weight (kg) used to express the answer in ml/kg·min (as above). The oxygen requirement for vertical work is:

$\dot{V}O_2$ in ml/kg·min = % grade* expressed as fraction × speed in m/min × 1.8 ml/kgm

EXAMPLE:

Question: What is the $\dot{V}O_2$ and MET level for an individual walking at 90 m/min (3.35 mph) up an incline of 13%?

Answer: Horizontal speed component:

$\dot{V}O_2$ in ml/kg·min = 90 m/min × 0.1 ml/kg·min per m/min + 3.5 ml/kg·min
= 12.5 ml/kg·min

Vertical work component:

$\dot{V}O_2$ in ml/kg·min = 0.13 × 90 m/min × 1.8 ml/kgm
= 21.1 ml/kg·min

Combining horizontal and vertical work:

$\dot{V}O_2$ in ml/kg·min = 12.5 ml/kg·min + 21.1 ml/kg·min
= 33.6 ml/kg·min
METS

---

*grade = fraction of vertical distance climbed per minute, divided by the belt speed.

$$= 33.6 \text{ ml/kg·min} \div 3.5$$
$$\text{ml/kg·min}$$
$$= 9.6$$

Question: You have two subjects who should exercise at 25.2 ml/kg·min or 7.2 METS to reach target heart rate. Subject A, because of an orthopedic problem, must walk no faster than 2 mph (54 m/min); subject B chooses to walk at 3.75 mph (100 m/min). At what grades do you set the treadmill for subjects A and B to reach a $\dot{V}O_2$ of 25.2 ml/kg·min?

Answer: Subject *A*
1. Horizontal component:
   $\dot{V}O_2$ in ml/kg·min = 54 m/min × 0.1 ml/kg·min per m/min + 3.5 ml/kg·min
   $$= 5.4 \text{ ml/kg·min} + 3.5 \text{ ml/kg·min}$$
   $$= 8.9 \text{ ml/kg·min}$$

2. Vertical component:
   Required $\dot{V}O_2$ minus $\dot{V}O_2$ of horizontal component = $\dot{V}O_2$ of vertical component.
   25.2 ml/kg·min − 8.9 ml/kg·min = 16.3 ml/kg·min
   16.3 ml/kg·min = % grade expressed as a fraction × 54 m/min × 1.8 ml/kgm
   Grade = 16.8%
   Subject *B*
1. Horizontal component:
   $\dot{V}O_2$ in ml/kg·min = 100 m/min × 0.1 ml/kg·min per m/min + 3.5 ml/kg·min
   $$= 13.5 \text{ ml/kg·min}$$

2. Vertical component:
Required $\dot{V}O_2$ minus $\dot{V}O_2$ of horizontal component = $\dot{V}O_2$ of vertical component
25.2 ml/kg·min − 13.5 ml/kg·min = 11.7 ml/kg·min
11.7 ml/kg·min = % grade expressed as a fraction × 100 m/min × 1.8 ml/kgm
Grade = 6.5%

Jogging/Running

A. Horizontal running for speeds exceeding 134 m/min (5 mph or 8 km/hr)
$\dot{V}O_2$ in ml/kg·min = speed in m/min × 0.2 ml/kg·min per m/min × kg body wt + 1 MET or 3.5 ml O_2/kg·min ÷ kg body wt
As in the equation for walking, body weight cancels out and the equation is reduced to:
$\dot{V}O_2$ in ml/kg·min = speed in m/min* × 0.2 ml/kg·min per m/min** + 3.5 ml/kg·min
EXAMPLE
Question: What $\dot{V}O_2$ and MET value is required to run on the flat at 200 m/min (7.5 mph)?
Answer: $\dot{V}O_2$ in ml/kg·min = 200 m/min × 0.2 ml/kg·min per m/min + 3.5 ml/kg·min

---

*For speeds in the units of km/hr (mph × 1.6 = km/hr) the MET requirement is approximately equal to the speed:
(10 km/hr = 10 METS; 12 km/hr = 12 METS or 6 mph = 1.6 × 6 = 9.6 METS).
**The energy requirement for running one meter/min = 0.2 ml/kg·min per m/min

$$= 43.5 \text{ ml/kg} \cdot \text{min} \div$$
$$3.5 \text{ ml/kg} \cdot \text{min (1}$$
MET)
$$= 12.4 \text{ METS}$$

Question: A subject has a $\dot{V}O_2$ max of 48 ml/kg·min. You wish him to run at a speed equal to 70% $\dot{V}O_2$ max. How fast should he run?

Answer: $0.70 \times 48 \text{ ml/kg} \cdot \text{min} = 33.6 \text{ ml/kg} \cdot \text{min}$

$$33.6 \text{ ml/kg} \cdot \text{min} = \text{speed in m/min} \times$$
$$0.2 \text{ ml/kg} \cdot \text{min per}$$
$$\text{m/min} + 3.5 \text{ ml/}$$
$$\text{kg} \cdot \text{min}$$

$$33.6 \text{ ml/kg} \cdot \text{min} -$$
$$3.5 \text{ ml/kg} \cdot \text{min} = 30.1 \text{ ml/kg} \cdot \text{min}$$

Divide the net $\dot{V}O_2$ (30.1 ml/kg·min) by the net energy requirement for running one meter/min (0.2 ml/kg·min per m/min). The units cancel; the answer is 150 m/min.

$$30.1 \text{ ml/kg} \cdot \text{min} \div 0.2 \text{ ml/kg} \cdot \text{min per m/min}$$
$$= 150 \text{ m/min}$$

or $\dfrac{150 \text{ m/min}}{26.8 \text{ m/min}} = 5.6$ mph

B. Inclined running at speeds exceeding 134 m/min.

For uphill running there is a difference in the oxygen requirements for running outdoors on solid ground or on a treadmill. Oxygen costs for running on the treadmill are lower than outdoors because the treadmill belt moves under the feet during the fraction of time the body is "airborne" when running (in contrast to walking when one foot is always on the ground).

As previously explained for walking, the estimation of the energy requirements for uphill jogging/running breaks down into the two components for horizontal speed and for the actually accomplished vertical work. The horizontal component, for both treadmill and outdoor running, is estimated as previously calculated: $\dot{V}O_2$ in ml/kg·min = speed in m/min × 0.2 ml/kg·min per m/min + 3.5 ml/kg·min

The oxygen costs for the actual vertical lift, to be added to the $\dot{V}O_2$ calculated for the horizontal component, are as follows:

For running outdoors:
$\dot{V}O_2$ in ml/kg·min = speed in m/min × % grade expressed as a fraction × 1.8 ml/kgm

For running uphill on the treadmill, the oxygen costs for the vertical component are approximately half the costs as for running outdoors on the same grade. Thus:
$\dot{V}O_2$ in ml/kg·min = speed in m/min × % grade expressed as a fraction × 1.8 ml/kgm × 0.5

EXAMPLE:

Question: What is the $\dot{V}O_2$ and the MET level for running at 180 m/min up a 5% grade?

Answer: A. Outdoors
$\dot{V}O_2$ in ml/kg·min = 180 m/min × 0.2 ml/kg·min per m/min + 1 MET (3.5 ml/kg·min)
= 39.5

Vertical component:
$\dot{V}O_2$ in ml/kg·min = 180 m/min × 0.05 × 1.8 ml/kgm
= 16.2

Total = 39.5 ml/kg·min + 16.2 ml/kg·min
= 55.7 ml/kg·min ÷ 3.5 ml/kg·min per MET
= 15.9 METS

   B. On a treadmill
       1. Horizontal component:
          Same as for outdoors.
       2. Vertical component:
          $\dot{V}O_2$ in ml/kg·min = 180 m/min ×
                              0.05 × 1.8
                              ml/kgm × .5
                          = 8.1 ml/kg· min
Total = 39.5 ml/kg·min + 8.1 ml/kg·min
      = 47.6 ml/kg·min ÷ 3.5 ml/kg·min per MET
      = 13.4 METS

Cycling: Bicycle Ergometer

The estimation of energy requirements for any form of cycling or cycle ergometry is different from that applied for walking, running, or stepping. The oxygen costs of cycling are almost entirely related to the set resistance, regardless of the individual's body weight. Thus, a person weighing 60 kg will have the same $\dot{V}O_2$ at a given work rate on the "bike" as a person weighing 90 kg. However, since the lighter person has a lower resting $\dot{V}O_2$, the relative energy expenditure, expressed in METS, is higher (METS = exercise $\dot{V}O_2$ ÷ resting $\dot{V}O_2$).

The work rate for cycle ergometer exercise is found by multiplying the force (kg of resistance) times the distance (m) through which the force acts, i.e., kg of resistance times the number of pedal revolutions (rpm) times the meters traveled per pedal revolution (kg × rpm × m = kgm). The kgm's are usually based on 50 rpm and 150 kgm/min = 25 watts. The energy requirement associated with cycle ergometer exercise is not only related to the set resistance in kgm, but includes internal or friction work and "static" muscle involvement counteracting the leg push. Consequently, there is an additional linear increase in energy demands with increasing exercise intensity. This additional work requires approximately a $\dot{V}O_2$ of 0.2 ml/kgm and is added to the 1.8 ml of $\dot{V}O_2$ needed for 1 kgm of work. Furthermore, to the thus estimated oxygen costs of the resistance work an average value of the $\dot{V}O_2$ at the resting position has to be added. This value for sitting cycle ergometry is approximately 300 ml.

The formula for estimating the oxygen demands for cycle ergometer exercise is:
$\dot{V}O_2$ in ml/min = work rate in kgm/min × 2 ml/kgm + sitting $\dot{V}O_2$ of 300 ml/min. This method provides reasonable estimates of the MET value for exercise intensities of 300 to 1200 kgm/min. Pedaling the ergometer against no resistance (zero load) requires approximately 550 ml O_2/min, or about 2 METS for a person of average body weight.

EXAMPLE:

One person weighing 60 kg and another weighing 75 kg are both performing exercise on the cycle ergometer set at a work rate of 900 kgm/min.

For both persons the:
$\dot{V}O_2$ in ml/kg·min = 900 kgm/min × 2 ml/kgm + 300 ml/min = 2100 ml/min

The relative energy costs for the 60 kg person are:
2100 ml/min ÷ 60 kg = 35 ml/kg·min, or:

35 ml/kg·min ÷ 3.5 ml/kg·min per MET = 10 METS
but for the 75 kg person: 2100 ml/min ÷ 75 kg = 28 ml/kg·min, or:

28 ml/kg·min ÷ 3.5 ml/kg·min per MET = 8 METS

Question: A patient, weighing 80 kg, must exercise at 5 METS on a bicycle ergometer to reach the target heart rate. At what work rate in kgm/min must you set the ergometer to demand this energy expenditure?

Answer: 5 METS = 5 (3.5 ml/kg·min) × 80 kg
            = 1400 ml/min.

$\dot{V}O_2$ in ml/min = kgm/min × 2 ml/kgm + 300 ml/min

1400 ml/min − 300 ml/min = 1100 ml/min
Divide the net cost of the work (1100 ml/min) by the net energy equivalent of 1 kgm of work (2 ml/kgm). The units cancel and the answer is 550 kgm/min.

1100 ml/min ÷ 2 ml/kgm = 550 kgm/min

Question: Assume that the above subject pedals the ergometer at 50 rpm and the wheel travels a distance of 6 m/rev. At what resistance, in kg, do you set the wheel to give 550 kgm/min?

Answer: kgm/min = resistance in kg force × distance moved per min in m/min

$$550 \text{ kgm/min} = ? \times \frac{50 \text{ rev}}{\text{min}} \times \frac{6 \text{ m}}{\text{rev}}$$

550 kgm/min = ? × 300 m/min

            = 1.8 kg

Stepping

The energy requirements for bench stepping vary with stepping rate and step height. The oxygen costs of stepping have been determined for the three components of vertical lift, stepping down, and stepping back and forth on a level surface.

The vertical work power production (lift work per unit time) is calculated from the stepping frequency and the height of the step (cm) as kgm/min. The oxygen costs for stepping up are:

$$kgm/min \times 1.8 \ ml/kgm$$

The oxygen costs for stepping down have been experimentally established to be one-third of the energy demands for stepping up. Thus, the combined $\dot{V}O_2$ for both stepping up and down is 1.33 times the $\dot{V}O_2$ for stepping up.

The energy costs for stepping back and forth on the level depend on the frequency of these movements. A simple estimation of these costs, in METS, is obtained by dividing the number of lifts per minute by 10.

For example: 30 lifts/min = 3 METS; 25 lifts/min = 2.5 METS, etc.

Below are a series of steps by which the $\dot{V}O_2$ and MET values for stepping can be calculated.

1. Determine the $\dot{V}O_2$ of stepping up and down.
$\dot{V}O_2$ in ml/min = height in m/lift × rate in lifts/min × 1.33 × 1.8 ml/kgm × kg body weight

2. To express the $\dot{V}O_2$ in ml/kg·min, divide the absolute $\dot{V}O_2$ by the body weight in kg.

3. Add the cost of stepping back and forth on the level. This can be estimated in METS by dividing the lifts per min by 10. For example, 30 lifts/min = 3 METS; 25 lifts/min = 2.5 METS, etc.

NOTE: The body weight entered in Step 2 above will cancel the body weight entered in Step 1. Consequently, the formula of Step 1 may be rewritten as follows:

$\dot{V}O_2$ in ml/kg·min = (ht in m/lift × rate in lifts/min × 1.33 × 1.8 ml/kgm) + $\dot{V}O_2$ of horizontal stepping.

EXAMPLE: 30 lifts/min

Question: What is the $\dot{V}O_2$ and MET level for a stepping frequency of 30 lifts/min if the bench height is 10 cm (0.1 m)?

Answer: $\dot{V}O_2$ in ml/kg·min = (0.1 m/lift × 30 lifts/min × 1.33 × 1.8 ml/kgm) + (10.5 ml/kg·min or 3 METS)

= (7.18 ml/kg·min + 10.5 ml/kg·min)

= 17.68 ml/kg·min ÷3.5 ml/kg·min per MET

= 5 METS

EXAMPLE: 24 lifts/min

Question: What is the $\dot{V}O_2$ and MET level for a stepping frequency of 24 lifts/min if the bench height is 24 cm (0.24 m)? (2.54 cm = 1 in)

Answer: $\dot{V}O_2$ in ml/kg·min $= (0.24$ m/lift $\times$ 24 lifts/min $\times$ 1.33 $\times$ 1.8 ml/kgm) + 8.4 ml/kg·min or 2.4 METS

$= (13.8$ ml/kg·min + 8.4 ml/kg·min)

$= 22.2$ ml/kg·min $\div 3.5$ ml/kg·min per MET

$= 6.3$ METS

Caution Regarding Environment

The energy requirements for walking, running, stepping, and cycling are relatively stable over a wide variety of environmental conditions. In contrast, the heart rate response associated with exercise will increase if the exercise is performed in hot or humid conditions or at altitude. As acclimatization is achieved the heart rate response will be reduced. Since safety is a basic concern when preparing appropriate exercise prescriptions, heart rate is probably the most useful guide in calculating the work of the heart and, hence, the exercise prescription. Thus, the heart rate prescription should accompany any prescription based on METS. Heart rate prescription is also of value when the calculation of METS is difficult, i.e., for activities that are intermittent in nature such as most sports and games.

Caution Regarding Rope Skipping

Rope skipping is one of the most frequently recommended exercises in aerobic training programs. The reasons are many. Rope skipping is an inexpensive rhythmical exercise that requires little space, can be done indoors or outdoors, and requires the expenditure of a large number of calories. The approximate energy requirement for skipping at 60 to 80 skips per minute is 9 METS and at 120 to 140 skips per minute is 11 to 12 METS. The heart rate response tends to be higher than expected at comparable MET levels for walking or running. The use of a small muscle mass in rope skipping may explain this difference in heart rate response.

In contrast to walking, running, stepping, or cycling, rope skipping cannot be considered a "graded" exercise in that the lowest rate of skipping (60 to 80 skips per minute) requires an energy expenditure close to the maximum METS found in the sedentary American population. In addition, doubling the rate of skipping requires an increase of only 2 to 3 METS. Therefore, caution should be used when recommending rope skipping for both symptomatic and asymptomatic participants.